KELLY, Pat

What you need to
know about breast cancer

What You Need to Know about Breast Cancer

Diagnosis, Treatment and Beyond

Sixth Edition

Pat Kelly, MA

Mark Levine, MD, MSc, FRCP(C)

KEY PORTER BOOKS

Library and Archives Canada Cataloguing in Publication

Kelly, Pat
    What you need to know about breast cancer : diagnosis, treatment and beyond / Pat Kelly ; with Mark Levine. — Rev. and updated 6th ed.

Includes index.

ISBN 1-55263-846-4

1. Breast—Cancer—Popular works. I. Levine, Mark N. II. Title.

RC280.B8K44 2006   616.99'449   C2006-902514-2

The publisher gratefully acknowledges the support of the Canada Council for the Arts and the Ontario Arts Council for its publishing program. We acknowledge the support of the Government of Ontario through the Ontario Media Development Corporation's Ontario Book Initiative.

We acknowledge the financial support of the Government of Canada through the Book Publishing Industry Development Program (BPIDP) for our publishing activities.

Key Porter Books Limited
Six Adelaide Street East, Tenth Floor
Toronto, Ontario
Canada M5C 1H6

www.keyporter.com

Text design: Jack Steiner
Electronic formatting: Jean Lightfoot Peters

Printed and bound in Canada

06 07 08 09 10 5 4 3 2 1

*As our readers face the challenges
that a cancer diagnosis can bring, we hope
that the knowledge of experienced caregivers,
the support of families and friends, and
the remembrance of all of the millions of
women now living after breast cancer
will bring hope and inspiration.*

From knowledge comes strength.

And

*To my daughters, Kate and
Kelly Fenn, who bring joy
and wisdom to my life.*

And to Chip—my dear anam cara—*friend of my soul.*

Acknowledgments

Once again, we are grateful to the many women living with breast cancer who helped make this book useful and supportive.

If you have any comments about this book, please address them to:

Pat Kelly
Email: pk@controlcancer.ca

Contents

Introduction

This book is for the thousands of women in both the United States and Canada who have been told, "I'm sorry, but you have breast cancer." It is also for the husbands, lovers, partners, friends, daughters, mothers, colleagues, co-workers, and family members who are trying to help and understand. This book has been written by experts in the field— women living with breast cancer and their doctors, people who know the journey from "the inside out."

The idea for this book began in 1988 in Burlington, Ontario, Canada. I had been diagnosed with breast cancer at the age of thirty-four and later met Barb Sullivan, who had been diagnosed a year earlier. Each of us was looking for support, information, and encouragement at a time when there were few breast cancer groups, information about treatments was very hard to find, and women didn't talk about cancer because they feared how others might react. Fortunately, Barb and I found each other and we soon realized there were probably other women like us looking for help, so we decided to hold a meeting. In April 1988, we first met at the local YMCA, where thirty-five women from our community joined us. Very quickly membership grew as other women came to share stories, to give support and information, to cry and to laugh, to mourn together for those who'd died and, most important, to learn to live *with* cancer. The group that started at the Y continues to meet every month, providing support, information, and advocacy for women and their families affected by breast cancer.

Much has happened since that first meeting. Women now talk openly about having cancer, information is easier to find, and survivors and advocates have made significant gains in the decision making about all aspects of the disease. All across Canada and the United States—from Fredericton to Detroit, from Thunder Bay to Washington—small groups have started with three or four women gathered at kitchen tables, in church basements, through Internet-based online Web sites and chat rooms, or in the waiting rooms of doctors' offices and clinics. More women are taking an active part in their diagnosis, treatment, and healing. Many groups and individuals are organizing advocacy efforts in order to bring about systemic changes in health care at the local, regional, and national levels.

While breast cancer continues to occur at alarmingly high rates, there is important good news. The death rate is finally starting to drop, moderately, in Canada and the United States, particularly in younger, premenopausal women. Clinical practice guidelines, outlining the best way to treat the disease, have now been developed as one way to ensure that all women and their doctors understand the range of options. Surgery, radiation, hormones, and chemotherapy are still standard treatment, but newer and more effective forms of some therapies are making a difference to survival rates. There is evidence that support groups, complementary therapies, and mind–body techniques, which encourage wellness, play an important role in the care and quality of life of women with breast cancer.

This sixth edition of our book was prompted by our readers' requests for both updated information about changes in treatment options and more discussion around the issues of recurrence and fears about death.

Medical research constantly produces new findings; it seems as soon as a book is published, new studies emerge that can change clinical practice. For these reasons we felt it was time to produce a revised edition of our book. As in the previous editions, we have tried to use the best evidence available to support the recommendations. The chapter on additional drug therapy after surgery has been updated to discuss the latest on the new drugs, trastuzumab and aromatase inhibitors. The chapter on recurrence of breast cancer discusses the additional therapies available since our last edition, and you will find expanded information about menopause, fertility, and sexuality.

Additionally, there has been an unprecedented explosion of information on the Internet. For women and their caregivers, who are searching for information, this is both a blessing and a curse. Consequently, we have expanded the resources section to include a more extensive listing of online resources, which will give readers a good place to start their research.

There has also been significant progress in influencing public policy around breast and other cancer research. Clearly, there is a link between the increase in advocacy and changes in government policy and funding for research, treatment, and cancer control programs. Without women's (and men's) tenacity and extraordinary fundraising talents, we doubt that research would have reached its present levels.

The relationship between us—once simply patient and doctor—has continued to grow in respect and value as we spend time and attention on our book. With this sixth edition, we have asked another breast cancer survivor and advocate—Beth Kapusta—to join our team. Beth brings a renewed energy and creativity to our efforts as a woman recently treated for this disease—and as a young, single mother and self-employed professional.

We hope our book reflects the heightened awareness about and needs of women now being diagnosed with breast cancer. Our intent is that this knowledge will serve to enlighten you—intellectually and spiritually—with honesty and compassion.

In hope and good health,
PAT KELLY AND MARK LEVINE
June 2006

Finding Out That You Have Breast Cancer

1

This chapter will help explain some of the most common emotional responses that women talk about when they learn they have breast cancer. It is intended to help you put these feelings into perspective and learn what other women have found helpful.

Illness is the night-side of life, a more onerous citizenship. Everyone who is born holds dual citizenship, in the kingdom of the well and in the kingdom of the sick. Although we all prefer to use only the good passport, sooner or later each of us is obliged, at least for a spell, to identify ourselves as citizens of that other place.

—SUSAN SONTAG,
Illness as Metaphor

I felt shocked...numb...and so angry at everyone...I hadn't done anything to deserve this...I kept hoping the doctors had made a mistake...

Many people remember very clearly the moment they heard their cancer diagnosis, but few of us remember anything else after hearing "it's cancer." Everything else is just noise.

There Must Be Some Mistake!

Few of us are ready when our fear of cancer becomes a reality. But each year more than 210,000 women in the United States and another 22,000 Canadian women learn that they have breast cancer. They are women of all ages and lifestyles; women who believed themselves to be healthy; women we know and care about; women just like us.

I was just thirty-four when I was diagnosed—and I was scared to death I would die. Not long after that, my husband and I divorced and I was alone with my two little girls. I remember those times as my "long, dark night of the soul." Last year, my oldest daughter graduated from university, the year before I earned a master's degree, and next year my youngest will earn her honors degree. I have a wonderful new partner and it will soon be twenty years since my diagnosis. I don't know if I could have been as conscious of these blessings, as grateful for my life, as willing to take risks, had my life not also been threatened by cancer. I am not saying cancer is a gift—it is a disease. But the gift came from learning that while I struggled, I realized that along with cancer came gratitude, awareness, and appreciation for the connectedness of human life.

Very few people truly understand what you're going through as a cancer patient. They care and they try to understand, but unless they've been there themselves, they really can't.

I think the most important goal is to provide those of us undergoing treatment with some hope that we will recover, survive, and perhaps even be cured. I am well enough aware of the severity of my illness not to fool myself that all is well. But the nurses, volunteers, and alternative practitioners that I have dealt with seem far more aware than my doctors of the power of language to affect empowerment in people.

If you have just learned that you have breast cancer, you could feel overwhelmed and unable to decide what to do next. You might be frightened. You might feel lonely. These feelings are very common for newly diagnosed women. *You are not alone. You are not helpless.* More than 2.5 million women living with breast cancer in North America prove these truths each and every day. There are people who can help you cope.

There is information that can help you make the right decisions for you. There is support for who you are now and what you must do.

Now might be a time to cry, to grieve, and to be angry. But it is also a time to care for yourself and learn more about breast cancer and its treatments. Soon you will be able to make decisions, plan your treatments, and begin to heal.

> One of the joys of surviving cancer has been the strengthened bond between myself and my husband and my children. We are kinder to each other now, realizing that there is no time for harsh words, no time to be wasted. Sometimes we cling together for a brief moment, sharing unspeakable thoughts in a terrifying yet richly comforting way.

As you begin to try to understand what it will be like to be treated for breast cancer, you might find it helpful to think about living with cancer as a journey. Like any other journey, you can plan but you cannot be certain where your trip will lead, when you will arrive, or what you will find along the way. The road ahead will be both good and bad. You will meet fellow travelers, learn to watch the view, tolerate the delays, and look forward to (or dread) the stops along the way.

You can begin your journey by replacing your fear about what might be ahead with information and support that you can use here and now.

> I was devastated and very sad. I realized that all the crap I had been ignoring needed looking at. I'm still on the journey and will always be recovering. After much counseling, marital and personal, my life is good. I'm learning to be real to others and myself. I'm listening to my body and respecting what it is telling me. I'm giving different messages to my three daughters—we are all feminists working to bring dignity, respect, and safety to all women, children, and men.

The Emotional Side of Cancer

When you learn that you have breast cancer, you can feel very alone or frightened. Some of us wonder if we are going crazy. We aren't. Cancer is a major life crisis. While you are in a crisis, you can expect to feel confused and emotional. Here are some of the emotions that breast cancer survivors remember from the time of their diagnosis and in the months that followed. Some of these feelings might be familiar to you.

> *Throughout my treatment, I felt I was being cared for quite well. My only complaint was that, other than a brief visit from a support group member, I felt very alone. If it weren't for my hospital roommate, it would have been terrifying. We have maintained our friendship and have a bond that no one who hasn't had cancer would have.*
>
> *It was tremendous—that experience of meeting other people with cancer for the first time! I just remember walking into the room, you know, somewhat nervous, not knowing who was going to be at that meeting. But I remember driving home afterward and just beaming because of walking into this room and meeting strangers and people I didn't know, but just to have this one big thing in common!*

FEAR

Fear of death. Fear of what life will be—can be—now. Fear of loss of strength, health, femininity, sexual attractiveness, and vigor. Fear of being diminished, of aging sooner than your time. Fear both for yourself and for your family and friends.

> *The initial diagnosis was traumatic for me. I was a thirty-six-year-old single parent. I was very scared. What would it be like? Was I going to*

die? After I got over the shock and everything settled down, the experience became very positive because it forced me to make changes in my life that I was putting off. I moved from where I was living, I made physical changes about how I looked, and I joined an exercise program. It made me realize how precious life is, and I'm much happier than I was before. When they did an ultrasound and thought the cancer had spread, I thought I was dying. But it hadn't. Now I'm just happy to be alive. Life is less scary when you have had cancer. Nothing is worse.

SHOCK AND DENIAL

You might be thinking, "This just can't be happening. I took good care of myself. I didn't smoke. I ate (mostly) healthy foods. I exercised. I handled the stress in my life. Nobody in my family has had breast cancer. So how could I have cancer?" The first reaction can be a temporary state of shock from which we gradually recuperate. When the initial feeling of numbness begins to disappear and we begin to collect our thoughts, the usual response is, "No, it can't be true." Since we all unconsciously think we are immortal, it is unimaginable to face the possibility of death. Fortunately, most women gradually adjust to the reality of diagnosis and decision making.

ANGER

Like many of us, you might be very angry that this disease has happened to you. Perhaps you found a lump or some change in your breast a while ago and didn't do anything about it. Or you discovered changes many months ago and your doctor said, "Let's just wait and see." Or you didn't go back to see your doctor. Now it's cancer. Anger at yourself or others is understandable and might be justifiable. But staying angry can also prevent you from making decisions or can get in the way of relationships with people you might need to depend on.

Finding ways to manage your anger will help you to cope with treatments and to communicate more effectively about your needs.

GUILT

Many women feel guilty about things that they did or didn't do and which they believe might have caused their cancer. *Always remember that you didn't do anything to cause the cancer.* The majority of women diagnosed with breast cancer have none of the known risk factors, other than age. There is probably no single cause of this disease. It just happened and no one can say for sure why it has happened to you. Learning to live with this uncertainty is one of the greatest challenges for women with breast cancer.

HOPELESSNESS/HELPLESSNESS

You might feel that your health is gone forever. You might even think your life is over. Overnight you have been transformed from a healthy, productive woman to someone you don't know, someone who is terribly ill and might, even now, be dying. You can feel hopeless and helpless, a cancer patient whose future is locked in place by this illness. You might, in your darkest moments, wish you could die quickly and painlessly right now and not have to face the uncertainty of the months ahead.

This sense of hopelessness is a common reaction. As you begin to gather information and meet the doctors and others who will care for you, you will realize that you are neither alone nor helpless—there are more than 2.5 million women in North America who are *living* with breast cancer. You, like many of us, might have difficulty adjusting to this shocking diagnosis, but the sense of helplessness will pass as you learn about this disease and its treatments. Remember that while no one can predict what will happen to *you*—the relative five-year survival rate for early stage breast cancer is more than 90 percent.

After my diagnosis, I had to stop working for the first time in my life. The debilitating treatments I was receiving made me dependent on my family and friends, which, being a very dynamic, active, and independent person, I had difficulty accepting.

ACCEPTING YOUR EMOTIONS

No one can say how long the ups and downs and the emotional grieving will continue. For some women, this period of uncertainty and confusion can last long after the end of their treatment.

I am envious of women who feel totally cured. I may not have cancer, but cancer certainly has me. I always feel like it's a lurking danger, like we're legally separated but can never be divorced. I live more on the edge now. I take risks that perhaps I shouldn't take and would never have taken before.

There will always be sadness for the losses, grief, and longing for what might have been a more carefree life. Those feelings eventually fade for most women. Cancer can be a turning point in your life. For now, try to remember that dramatic mood swings are to be expected. They are part of learning to be a cancer survivor. You might keep coming back to these emotions as you learn to live with cancer and go from being a patient to a woman whose life has been challenged by cancer.

I wonder if I will ever make plans again?

Life goes on around me. I am aware of it but not involved. I am unto myself. Tears are close, always.

Today I need to work. To have another identity besides "patient." I am tired. But I must fight. Say no to this intrusion. Not lay down my will.

This is the last exercise class with a real breast. Next time I'll have to worry about my socks falling out.

How do you say goodbye to a breast? I've had it for forty-five years. I think I'll miss it. But I'm playing it cool.

The cancer lady comes. Shows me her wares. Great flopping prosthesis. I think yuck! I am not interested right now. She says, "Don't carry your purse on your affected side and always wear your gloves when gardening!" May she strangle in her knickers.

It is more complicated than I thought. I wasn't going to be bothered by losing a breast. I am. I don't like how I look. I look amputated. I am different. I am a cancer patient. Will I ever be unaware of my chest?

Did you know you can't cry while lying on your back? You get water in your ears.

A large sign says Cancer Clinic. I am identified even before I enter. I want to go in disguise. I do not belong here. I think I will leave.

It is a sit-on-the-edge-of-your-seat kind of place. Scary. At the mercy of machines. All supposed to do a job. But do they?

Tell me again that I'll be fine. Give me hope to grow with. Words to recover by.

—BARB SULLIVAN,
My Broken Breast Book

Start by Helping Yourself—Two Decisions for People with Cancer

There are two questions you might consider asking yourself about how you choose to cope with your diagnosis: first, "Will I be passive or active?" Being passive means doing what you are told to do about diagnosis and treatment and otherwise just trying to forget this ever happened. Being active means learning, asking questions, taking responsibility for yourself, your decisions, and your recovery.

The second question you might then ask is, "What can I do to help myself to cope, to heal, to grow, and to learn to live fully?"

The most basic skill in managing your emotional response to cancer is deep relaxation. Not the kind of relaxation "quick-fix" that comes with a glass of wine and TV, but relaxation that involves learning to recognize tension in your body and learning to let it go. It's a simple, learned skill that can become an important tool for helping you get through waiting times in the cancer clinic, waiting for lab results, getting back to sleep at 3 a.m., adjusting to the changes in your body, struggling to find a way to talk to kids, friends, employers. Learning coping skills NOW can make this time much easier for you—and it can become a lifelong practice in self-care. *Healing Journey: Using Your Mind to Foster a Healing Environment in Your Body,* a book and CD set by Dr. Alastair Cunningham, is an excellent self-directed learning program. There are many other valuable resources—books, CDs, groups, audiotapes that can help you learn basic techniques in stress management, relaxation response, and positive mental imaging. You might also look for help through the Center for Mind-Body Medicine at www.cmbm.org. The center is a nonprofit, educational organization dedicated to a model of medicine that combines the precision of modern science with the wisdom of ancient healing. It addresses the mental, emotional, social, and spiritual, as well as physical, dimensions of health and illness.

At the very least, learning these simple techniques will help you feel more relaxed, more in control, and help you to think clearly even at the most difficult times.

WHAT OTHER KINDS OF HELP ARE AVAILABLE?

> ... all humans are frightened of our own solitude. Yet only in solitude can we learn to know ourselves and learn to handle our own eternity of aloneness.
>
> —HAN SUYIN

Many kinds of help are available to deal with the emotional burden you or your family members can feel. Beginning with your own circle of connections—to friends, family, spiritual and religious communities, colleagues and co-workers—the people with whom you have established relationships might be ready, willing, and able to offer emotional and practical support. Equally, they might need some signal from you that you are ready to receive that help.

A recent poll of 1,000 people living with cancer in the United States from the Lance Armstrong Foundation found that 78 percent of respondents did not seek the services of a counselor, social worker, or psychologist. People living with cancer often lack the resources for the emotional support that may be available through family, friends, professionals, and cancer centers.

You might consider asking the people at your local cancer center what support services are available. Many cancer centers employ professionals in the area of psychosocial oncology or patient and caregiver support. These people specialize in cancer care and are concerned with understanding and treating the social, psychological, emotional, spiritual, and practical aspects of cancer.

Psychosocial oncology professionals are there to help you with your fears and strong emotions. They are specially trained to deal with cancer patients and their loved ones because the physical effects of cancer are uniquely difficult and nearly impossible to separate from the emotional distress they cause. They are experienced in helping you with self-esteem and body issues often associated with the scarring caused by surgical treatments for breast cancer. For example, these professionals offer help to people living on their own, those whose first language is not English, recent immigrants, children and elderly people, gays and lesbians, as well as people who have other health challenges in addition to having cancer.

Another key role these counselors play is as problem-solving guides or "navigators." This includes helping patients and families find and manage information, acting as a gateway to personalized needs, such as support groups, financial resources, books and information. Many cancer patients find that the overwhelming quantity of information in some areas can be just as daunting as the lack of information in others (particularly in hard-to-talk-about areas such as fertility, sexuality, and cancer). Counselors are knowledgeable about what information is available, and can help you determine which additional information you might need and when. For instance, they can direct young mothers to information on how to talk to their children about breast cancer, or find information about preserving fertility after treatment, transportation to treatments, and so on.

Counselors are also experienced in helping patients and families with practical issues, such as financial and insurance resources. They can give you a sense of what financial help might be available, and help you fill out forms.

TYPES OF COUNSELING

Counseling is part of an integrated team approach to treating patients' needs in a holistic way. A holistic approach pays attention to the needs of the "whole person"—physical, mental, social, and spiritual. Different individuals might be available for counseling, depending on the services in your community and your level of need. Most cancer centers offer individual counseling by psychologists, psychiatrists, social workers, and chaplains, as well as pain and symptom management nurses, dieticians, and physician specialists.

While counselors do much of their work one-on-one with patients, they also work with families. Some departments offer group counseling or peer support groups led by a trained professional.

SUPPORT GROUPS

> *My weekly, professionally led support group meetings are so valuable at keeping life in perspective. We talk about everything in a very candid way—our kids, our sex lives (or lack of them), our coping techniques, our ways of trying to get control of our lives back, and our deepest, darkest fears. The last one is probably the most important: while I'm lucky to have a supportive partner, I feel that sharing all of my darkest thoughts with him is an unfair burden. With the girls, we are all letting these demons out together and somehow this makes them more manageable.*

Many women find that support groups are very helpful in dealing with the emotional side of cancer. At a support group you can expect to meet other women who are living with breast cancer. Some members are newly diagnosed; others will still be coming to the group years after their treatments have ended. You can talk about your fears or relationships, or you might just want to sit quietly and listen. But, most important, you meet other women who know about living with breast cancer. Support groups can offer support and education, even laughter and warmth, along with hope. In groups, participants talk about their fears about death or pain, relationships with family, friends, and doctors, coping with treatment and side effects, complementary and alternative therapies, financial and insurance problems.

People who participate in support groups talk about helping one another in four ways:

1. by listening and telling one another their stories
2. by sharing information, practical tips, and experiences
3. by offering nonjudgmental emotional support and modeling coping skills
4. by creating a sense of belonging to the group.

Support groups aren't for everyone; in fact, many women find all the comfort and support they need among friends and family. Again, consider groups as one option to explore, not a requirement for everyone.

ASSESSING YOUR EMOTIONAL STATUS

Emotional distress, anxiety, and even depression are very common experiences for many women when they are diagnosed with breast cancer—in fact, 35 to 45 percent of breast cancer patients experience these symptoms at some point during their cancer journey. Reaching out for help can be a difficult step, but it can make the difference between a long and lonely time and a period of gaining hope and help from others.

The following questionnaire can help you determine whether you might be suffering from emotional distress and could benefit from professional counseling. Everyone experiences some of these symptoms at some time during their lifetimes; there are no right or wrong answers. Take some time to fill out the questionnaire and consider talking with a professional about your support options.

PATIENT SELF-ASSESSMENT QUESTIONNAIRE

During the past two weeks:

1. I have felt anxious or worried about cancer and the treatment I am receiving.

1	2	3	4	5
Not at all				All the time

2. I have felt depressed or discouraged.

1	2	3	4	5
Not at all				All the time

3. I have been irritable or unusually angry and I have not controlled it well.

1	2	3	4	5
Not at all				All the time

4. My sleeping habits have changed.

1	2	3	4	5
Not at all				Very much

5. I have experienced a change in my appetite.

1	2	3	4	5
Not at all				Very much

6. I have had difficulty concentrating at work or at home, or on routine things such as reading the newspaper or watching television.

1	2	3	4	5
Not at all				Very much

7. Cancer and its treatment have interfered with my daily activities.

1	2	3	4	5
Not at all				Very much

8. Cancer and its treatment have interfered with my family or social life.

1	2	3	4	5
Not at all				Very much

9. Cancer and its treatment have interfered with my sexual life.

1	2	3	4	5
Not at all				Very much

10. Pain and discomfort have caused me to limit my activities.

1	2	3	4	5
Not at all				Very much

11. Cancer has caused physical, emotional, or financial hardship for me.

1	2	3	4	5
Not at all				Very much

12. Cancer and its treatment have caused changes in my physical appearance and this concerns me.

1	2	3	4	5
Not at all				Very much

13. I have had difficulty coping with the stress I have experienced.

1	2	3	4	5
Not at all				Very much

11. My quality of life during the past two weeks has been:

1	2	3	4	5
Excellent				Very poor

If you find that many of your answers are in columns four or five, you could be experiencing significant distress and you might consider discussing your feelings with a counselor.

This chart was developed by and used with permission from Beth Kapusta with the Canadian Association of Psychosocial Oncology for The

Emotional Facts of Life with Cancer, and based on tools developed by the Tom Baker Cancer Centre Department of Psychosocial Resources and Northwestern Ontario Regional Cancer Centre Supportive Care Program.

SUMMARY

As you will have realized by now, cancer is as much an emotional and psychological experience as it is physical. Feeling hurt, angry, or confused is normal. There are many different ways of dealing with the emotional distress, but don't feel that you have to manage everything alone. Reaching out, whether to the support staff of your treatment center, or to the family and friends who might share some of these worries and feelings with you, is important for your healing process. Everyone who cares about you will be looking to you to give them a signal; let them know if you want to talk (or don't want to talk) and how they can help.

Only after I had made my treatment choice and completed my radiation did I decide to participate in a support group. The group was fantastic in terms of sharing information, articles, videos, personal experiences, and doctors' names. I wish I had gone sooner. But I just felt I could handle things on my own and that the group was more of a "psychological thing" for people who were having trouble handling their diagnosis. I think doctors should encourage patients to participate.

Remember that you have control over the choices you make and *how* you choose to make this journey through cancer territory. Like many other women, you might also find meaningful and rewarding surprises along the way to healing.

Beauty and tragedy are inextricably interwoven in people with serious illness. Those with diseases such as cancer can be heroic and frightened, generous and selfish. They can indeed "live beyond limits."

—DR. DAVID SPIEGEL,
*Living Beyond Limits: New Hope
and Help for Facing Life-Threatening Illness*

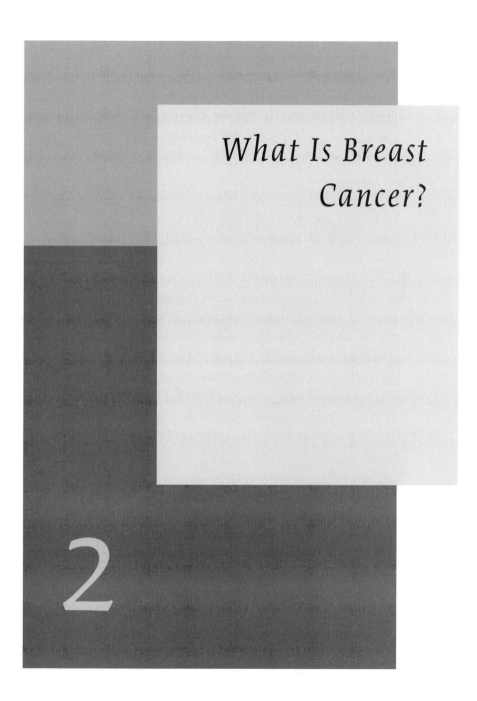

What Is Breast Cancer?

2

This chapter will explain what breast cancer is. It will also explore some of the risk factors for breast cancer, and why some women are more likely to get it than others. As you will see, risk factors really don't help explain why most women develop breast cancer. There is still much that is unknown about the cause of this disease.

Cancer's just a word—not a sentence.

—HANNA HEIDE

There is both a blessing and a burden to being a modern-day cancer patient. A generation ago, patients argued for more information, more choice, and more input about their treatment. To a great extent, that is what we have received—but with all this information and choice, there often comes overwhelming uncertainty. People want to feel that they are a part of their health care team, but they don't want to be abandoned to make decisions on their own. The information in this chapter is intended to help you understand more about the types of breast cancer and diagnostic tests.

The surgeon saw me on Thursday and advised an immediate mastectomy, which I had the following day. He was kindness personified and I was sure he was right. I felt a tremendous sense of urgency to "get on" with my surgery. Looking back on the good and bad aspects of my personal experience, being advised to have immediate surgery was GOOD, but I wish I had taken more time to consider my options.

A Life-Changing Disease

While it is often thought of as a single disease, cancer is actually a group of more than 100 different diseases characterized by the uncontrolled abnormal growth of cells that can spread throughout the body. Cancer begins when normal cells live beyond their normal life cycle, enabling them to continue to divide and reproduce uncontrollably, crowding out normal cells. Most cancers form a lump or mass called a tumor. Tumors can be made of noncancerous cells and are called benign. Benign tumors do not grow uncontrollably and are not life-threatening. Cancerous tumors are called malignant and they can invade and destroy healthy tissue. They can also release cells that break away and travel to other parts of the body where they continue to grow. This spreading is called metastasis. When cancer spreads, it is still named for the part of the body where it started. For example, if breast cancer spreads to the lungs it is still called breast cancer, not lung cancer.

HOW DOES BREAST CANCER START?

Like all forms of cancer, breast cancer starts in one cell. Cells are the smallest structural unit of living matter that can function independently in the body. They are the building blocks of our bodies. Healthy cells grow at a normal rate. Cancer cells grow at an accelerated rate and continue to grow until they crowd out the normal cells. Unlike normal cells, cancer cells don't know how to turn off their growth. The abnormal growth rate is caused by changes or mutations in the genetic material inside the cell. These mutations can be inherited from our parents or caused by being exposed to a mutating substance. It usually takes more than one "hit" of exposure to a cancer-causing substance to cause changes. Cancerous tumors or lumps contain both normal cells and mutated cells.

IS ALL BREAST CANCER THE SAME?

In a word, no. There are several kinds of breast cancer, depending on where in the breast tissue the tumor starts to grow. About one-half of all breast cancer tumors are first found in the upper, outer part of the breast, but they can appear anywhere in the breast tissue. Each breast has fifteen to twenty sections, called "lobes," which have many smaller sections, called "lobules." Thin tubes, called "ducts," connect the lobes and lobules. The lobes, lobules, and ducts make and secrete milk for breast-feeding. Eighty-five percent of breast cancers start in the ducts, 12 percent in the lobules, and the remaining 2 percent start in the surrounding tissue. Not all breast cancers are found in the form of a lump. Other changes that can indicate cancer are dimpling around the nipple, secretions or fluid leaking from the nipple, and changes in the skin texture that may make it look like the skin of an orange, called "peau d'orange."

Carcinoma in Situ (CIS)

"In situ" means the cancer is confined to the ducts or lobules and has not spread to the surrounding fatty tissue.

Lobular Carcinoma in Situ (LCIS)

This form of cancer begins in the lobules but does not spread through their walls. Most cancer specialists believe that LCIS does not develop into invasive cancer, but women with LCIS are at a higher risk of developing other kinds of breast cancer in both the same and opposite breast.

Ductal Carcinoma in Situ (DCIS)

This is a very common type of non-invasive tumor that does not spread outside the duct walls. Some specialists think more women die *with* DCIS than *because* of it. Thirty years ago DCIS was diagnosed in about

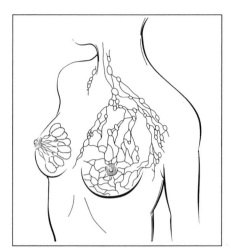

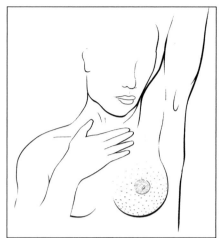

FIGURE 2.1 *Cross-section of breast showing the network of milk-producing lobes connected by thin tubes or ducts*

FIGURE 2.2 *Inflammatory breast cancer (peau d'orange)*

6 percent of patients. Today, about 20 percent of patients are diagnosed with DCIS, probably due to advances in early detection through mammography. Treatment is usually surgery and radiation.

Infiltrating Lobular Carcinoma (ILC)

Lobular carcinoma starts in the lobes of the breast and, like ductal carcinoma, it can spread to other parts of the body through blood or the lymph system. About 12 percent of breast cancers start in the lobules or lobes.

Infiltrating Ductal Carcinoma (IDC)

This type of breast cancer starts inside the cells of the milk ducts and invades outside the duct walls into the surrounding tissue. Over time, it can also spread through the lymph system or bloodstream to other organs or bones. Infiltrating ductal carcinoma accounts for about 85 percent of all breast cancers.

Inflammatory Breast Cancer (IBC)

This is an uncommon type of breast cancer that can cause redness, swelling, and an increase in skin temperature. The cancer cells in inflammatory breast cancer are located in the lymph vessels of the skin, growing in sheets rather than as a solid tumor. It can often be found spread throughout the breast with no solid tumor or palpable mass. There can be increased breast density compared with previous mammograms, which should be considered a suspicious finding. One or more of the following symptoms can be caused by IBC:

- Swelling, itching, bruising, or thickening of skin, usually sudden, sometimes a cup size in a few days
- Pink, red, or dark-colored area of skin, sometimes textured like an orange (peau d'orange)
- Nipple retraction, discharge, or change in color and texture
- Breast is hot or warm to the touch
- Breast pain (throbbing, constant ache to stabbing pains)

Paget's Disease

Paget's disease shows up as itching and scaling of the nipple that doesn't get better. It is a form of DCIS. Sometimes there is cancer inside the breast tissue as well.

HOW DOES CANCER SPREAD OUTSIDE THE BREAST?

Cancer cells can break off from the tumor and travel through blood vessels or lymph fluid to other organs and bones. When you are diagnosed with breast cancer, and before you begin treatment, your doctors will examine you and perform tests, X-rays, and scans that will help to determine if your cancer has spread beyond the breast to lymph tissue or to other organs.

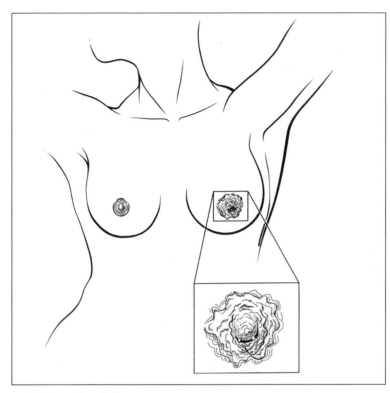

FIGURE 2.3   *Paget's disease*

HOW FAST DOES BREAST CANCER GROW?

Some cancers grow quickly, while others grow slowly—growing, resting, and then growing again. How fast a tumor grows varies from one person to the next. Although it can be difficult to wait for your test results so you can make treatment decisions, you do have time to learn about your type of breast cancer and carefully consider which options will be best for you. The average doubling time of a breast cell is 100 days. It takes approximately a billion cells to form a breast tumor 1 cm in size, which means that, on average, most cancers have been around for six to ten years before they can be felt as a lump or seen on a mammogram.

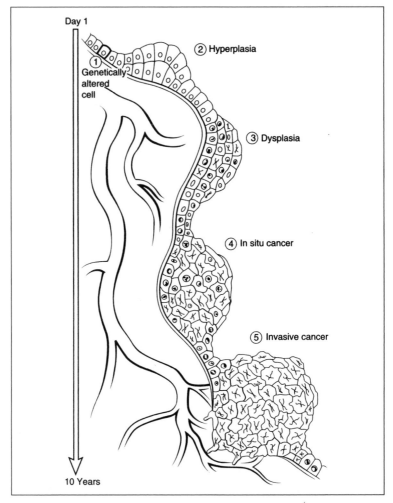

Day 1

① Genetically altered cell

② Hyperplasia

③ Dysplasia

④ In situ cancer

⑤ Invasive cancer

10 Years

FIGURE 2.4   *Progression from a single cell change to tumor mass (please refer to Glossary for explanation of terms)*

WHY IS CANCER SO HARD TO TREAT OR CURE?

Cancer is not something that invades our body from the outside like a virus or bacteria; cancer is not like an injury or trauma. Cancer is a disease of the self: the body's own cells change and grow out of control.

WHAT IS BREAST CANCER?

Another problem is that cancer cells are often very "smart" and find ways to resist treatments. This is why it is so hard to stop cancer cells from growing without also harming healthy cells.

> *Our main goal in society should be to find a way to kill cancer cells. All money should go to this goal, since with a cure, the need for many other services would be eliminated. Effective research is the key to a cure for cancer. We can put people on the moon—why can't we kill a cancer cell?*

SHOULD I GET A SECOND OPINION?

"You'll have to convince me you know what you're doing," I said.

"Look, I've done a large number of these. I've never had anyone die, and I've never made anyone worse."

"Yeah, but why should you be the person who operates on me?"

"Because as good as you are at cycling"—he paused—"I'm a lot better at brain surgery."

—LANCE ARMSTRONG, *It's Not about the Bike*

Dr. Susan Love, a U.S. surgeon and breast cancer activist, has stated, "Sometimes patients are shy about seeking second opinions—as though they're somehow insulting their doctor's professionalism. Never feel that way. You're not insulting us; you're simply seeking the most precise information possible in what may literally be a life-and-death situation. Most doctors won't be offended and if you run into a doctor who does get miffed, don't be intimidated. Your life and your peace of mind are more important than your doctor's ego."

My surgeon seemed to be looking at me from a great height. He was
openly angry when I sought out the cancer clinic for a second opinion.

You might want to ask your family doctor or specialist to refer you for a second opinion if you feel uncomfortable or need more information about the options being suggested to you. For women in remote and rural areas, you might have to travel to get a second opinion. Only you can determine how necessary this is for you. If you know other women who have had breast cancer, ask them how they were treated and who their specialists were. To find other breast cancer patients you can talk to, or to find out about services and support groups in your area, see the Resources section at the back of this book.

You alone know your body. You alone know when you're not feeling right. Ask questions and feel worthy. If you get unsatisfactory answers, get second, third, and fourth opinions....Demand answers.

—JACKI RALPH JAMIESON, *singer-songwriter*

There are still many unanswered questions in the field of breast cancer research. There might not be just one answer or even a "right" answer to some of the questions you will have. Ask around. Talk to family and friends. Get as much information as you need before making any decisions.

> Women are overwhelmed, distraught, when the diagnosis of cancer is confirmed. It is difficult at such a time to process all sorts of new and very technical facts. It is not a time when people should be pressured to make quick decisions overnight.
>
> —DR. KAREN GELMAN

There are many sources of good information. In the U.S., the American Cancer Society (www.cancer.org), the American Society for Clinical Oncology (www.asco.org), and the National Cancer Institute's Web sites are thorough and informative (see Resources section). If you are in Canada, you might find it helpful to read "Canadian Clinical Practice Guidelines for the Care and Treatment of Breast Cancer," published by the *Canadian Medical Association Journal* (CMAJ). Copies of the guidelines are available by calling the Cancer Information Service at 1-888-939-3333 or on the Web at www.breastcancerguide.ca.

I had a very bad experience with my surgeon and hope in future women know they can ask for second opinions and not feel guilty. It was only by accident that I spoke with an oncologist and radiologist and learned that I had had an option other than the mastectomy.

At the time of printing this book, a network of support groups for women with breast cancer is flourishing across the United States and Canada. Some individual states, regions, and provinces have their own support network as well. If you are having difficulty connecting with a support group, contact your local office of the American Cancer Society or Canadian Cancer Society. You will also find information about support groups in the Resources section of this book.

Remember too that there are many other places to find support:

among your family and friends, family doctor, nurses, and co-workers. They could be waiting for a sign that you want to talk—or be struggling to know what to do. You might want to ask a friend or family member to read this book along with you. People want to help, but you need to let them know what you need from them and when you need it.

Who Gets Breast Cancer?

This section will explain some of the risk factors for breast cancer, and why some women are more likely to get it than others. As you will see, risk factors really don't explain why some women develop breast cancer. Much is still unknown about the causes of this disease.

WHY DID THIS HAPPEN TO ME?

What is the most important breast cancer risk factor? Simply being a woman.

Many women who have just learned of their condition wonder what they might have done to cause the disease. No one can tell you exactly what caused your body to develop breast cancer. The known risk factors are not very helpful in understanding why some women get the disease. Not everyone who has a high risk will get breast cancer. Many women who are diagnosed have none of the risk factors. The effects of risk factors are modest at best.

RISKS FOR DEVELOPING BREAST CANCER

Scientific researchers have identified some factors that increase a woman's risk of breast cancer. Having breast implants to change your breast size or shape, or to rebuild a breast after surgery, has not been found to be a risk factor for breast cancer. Factors that have been consistently found to increase risk include:

- Age: risk increases as you get older
- Personal and family history/genetics: having a close relative(s) with breast cancer
- Gender: More than 99 percent of breast cancers occur in women
- Previous exposure to breast radiation: exposure of the breast to high levels of ionization radiation (i.e., X-rays) or lower levels before age two
- Obesity: being overweight/obese (only after menopause), based on your Body Mass Index (BMI)

Reproductive history
- Having a first baby after age thirty or never having a baby
- Age at the start of your first period: early menstruation (before age twelve)
- Age at the start of your menopause: late menopause (after age fifty-five)
- HRT: taking hormone replacement therapy
- Never breast-feeding

Factors that have been less consistently found to increase breast cancer risk include:

- Drinking alcohol
- Being physically inactive
- Smoking tobacco
- Using birth control pills. Note that although taking birth control pills appear to slightly increase a woman's risk of breast cancer, the risk of ovarian cancer is decreased.

Simply because we are women, and our bodies produce hormones and we develop breasts, we are all at risk for breast cancer. There is also a risk for men, though it is much smaller: about 1 in every 100 breast cancer cases are diagnosed in men.

Seventy percent of women with breast cancer have none of the known risk factors, other than age. Risk factors are based on the information and statistics gathered from large groups of women. Other than inherited gene mutations, the effect of any specific risk factor for any individual woman is small. Even when your risk factors are known, no one can predict what will happen to any one woman in particular.

THE CAUSES OF BREAST CANCER

There is probably no single cause of this disease. Researchers have found that several different factors working together appear to increase the risk of breast cancer. The ways in which different risk factors interact with each other is not fully understood. Because of their genetic history, their lifestyles, and what they are exposed to in their lifetime, some women are more likely to get the disease than others. The incidence of breast cancer is higher in industrialized countries, such as Canada, Northern Europe, and the United States, than in other parts of the world.

The following information about risk factors provides some further explanations.

RISK FACTORS YOU CANNOT CHANGE

Age

The risk of developing breast cancer increases as a woman grows older. Two-thirds of breast cancers are diagnosed in women over the age of fifty.

The chance of a woman having invasive breast cancer some time during her life is about 1 in 8. Breast cancer death rates are going down. This decline is probably the result of finding the cancer earlier and improved treatment

	Within Two Years	Within Five Years	Within Ten Years
Age, Year			
35	0.08	0.26	0.74
40	0.16	0.48	1.25
45	0.29	0.78	1.68
50	0.36	0.92	1.95
55	0.40	1.06	2.30
60	0.50	1.29	2.65
65	0.57	1.43	2.86
70	0.62	1.54	2.97

TABLE 1: PROBABILITY OF MANIFESTING BREAST CANCER (%)

SOURCE: *Used with permission from the* Canadian Medical Association Journal, *1994*

Personal and Family History/Genetics

If you have already had breast cancer, or a close family member was diagnosed with breast cancer before they reached menopause, you are at greater risk. For example, if your mother had breast cancer before age forty, your risk of developing this disease is doubled. And if you have many other close relatives with breast cancer, your risk could be much higher.

Recent research shows that some women with breast cancer have inherited a mutated gene linked to the development of breast cancer (BRCA2) or breast and ovarian cancer (BRCA1). Factors that should alert you to the possibility of either mutant gene being present include: early onset of disease (before age thirty-five), family history (on either side) of diagnoses in every generation, a male family member with breast cancer, and linkage with ovarian cancer.

However, if both you and a close family member develop breast cancer, it is not necessarily because the same gene is present. The field of research on genetics and breast cancer is relatively new. Discoveries are being made quite rapidly in the area.

A mutant BRCA1 gene on chromosome 17 is probably responsible for about 2 percent of the breast cancer cases diagnosed each year. As many as one-quarter of these cases, in Canada and the U.S., occur in women aged forty-five and younger. A mutant BRCA1 gene is found in nearly half of the families with a high incidence of breast cancer and in at least 80 percent of the families with a history of both early onset breast cancer and ovarian cancer.

There are several options available for women with BRCA1 or BRCA2 inherited mutations. Surgical options include prophylactic mastectomy (removal of the breasts), and oophrectomy (removal of the ovaries). The drug tamoxifen has been used for many years as a treatment for some types of breast cancer. Recent studies show that women at high risk for breast cancer are less likely to get the disease if they take tamoxifen. Another drug, raloxifene, is also being studied for use in reducing breast cancer risk and appears to be as good as tamoxifen. And there are even newer drugs now under study.

If you have been diagnosed with breast cancer and your age or family history suggests that the BRCA1 or BRCA2 gene might be present, your doctor should refer you to a genetics specialist. This could have an impact on your treatment and also on other family members. For example, if you have the abnormal gene, mastectomy might be a better option rather than lumpectomy and radiation because there may be other tumors in your breast. On the other hand, there is so much going on with the recent diagnosis of breast cancer, it could be better for you to first have the surgery and postoperative radiation therapy. When this treatment is finished, you can then see the genetics specialist and be tested for BRCA1/2. At this time, there will be less on your mind and you will be able to focus on the many issues involved.

Preventive (Prophylactic) Mastectomy for Women with Very High Breast Cancer Risk

For the few women who are at very high risk for breast cancer, prophylactic mastectomy can be an option. The purpose of the surgery is to reduce the risk by removing both breasts before breast cancer is diagnosed. The reasons for considering this type of surgery may include one or more of the following risk factors:

+ mutated BRCA genes found by genetic testing
+ previous cancer in one breast, strong family history (breast cancer in several close relatives)
+ biopsy specimens showing lobular carcinoma in situ (LCIS)

Before considering a prophylactic mastectomy, discuss this option with a specialist (e.g., your oncologist or a genetics specialist). There is no way to know ahead of time how this surgery will affect a particular woman. Some women with BRCA mutations will develop a fatal breast cancer early in life, and a prophylactic mastectomy before the cancer occurs might add many years to their life expectancy. Although most women with BRCA mutations develop breast cancer, some don't, and these women would not benefit from the surgery.

It is also important to realize that while a prophylactic mastectomy removes nearly all of the breast tissue, a small amount remains. So although this operation markedly reduces the risk of breast cancer, a cancer can still develop in the breast tissue that remains attached to the skin after surgery. So far, this has been a rare problem.

Although women might develop breast cancer that can be found by mammography or breast exam and be treated by mastectomy,

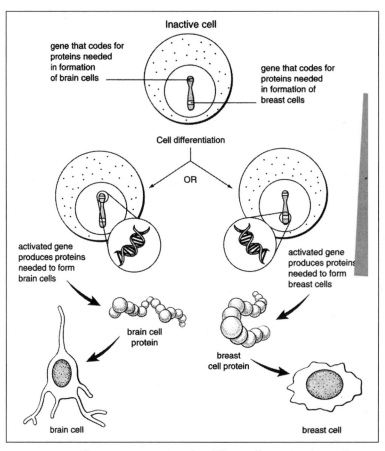

Inactive cell

gene that codes for proteins needed in formation of brain cells

gene that codes for proteins needed in formation of breast cells

Cell differentiation

OR

activated gene produces proteins needed to form brain cells

activated gene produces proteins needed to form breast cells

brain cell protein

breast cell protein

brain cell

breast cell

FIGURE 2.5 *Different genes are activated in different cells, creating the specific proteins that program a particular type of cell to develop.*

these women still face a high risk of cancer in the remaining breast. Some women with BRCA mutations who have had a breast cancer in one breast and who do not wish to have a prophylactic mastectomy are being followed by annual MRI of the breast. Second opinions are strongly recommended before any woman makes the decision to have this surgery. The American Cancer Society board of directors has stated that, "Only very strong clinical and/or pathologic indications warrant doing this type of preventive operation." Nonetheless, after careful consideration, this might be the right choice for some women.

Although this book is not about ovarian cancer, it is important that women with a BRCA mutation recognize they have a high risk of developing ovarian cancer. Most doctors recommend that the ovaries be surgically removed once childbearing is complete. None of these procedures—alone or in combination—completely eliminates the risk of breast cancer, so women at genetic risk need to make sure that close medical follow-ups are part of their health regime. There are now genetic counselors and oncologists with special expertise in managing BRCA-associated breast cancer.

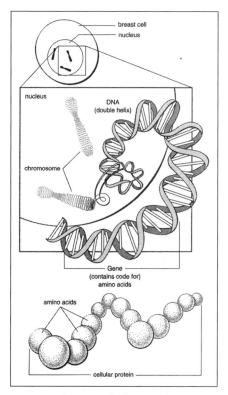

FIGURE 2.6   *DNA, which carries the instructions that allow cells to make proteins, is made up of four chemical bases. Tightly coiled strands of DNA are packaged in units called chromosomes, housed in the cell's nucleus. Working subunits of DNA are known as genes.*

Most diseases and traits don't follow simple patterns of inheritance; a variety of factors influence how a gene will perform. Genes come in pairs, with one part inherited from each parent. The BRCA1 susceptibility gene can be inherited from either parent. But even if you have this gene, your risk of disease by age sixty-five is 60 percent, not 100 percent.

There are counseling programs available for anyone who might have an inherited risk for cancer, and your family doctor should be able to tell you where your nearest counseling center is located. You can also contact the American Cancer Society (1-800-ACS-2345) or, in Canada, the Cancer Information Service (1-888-939-3333) and inquire about your local services.

Previous Exposure to Breast Radiation

Women who as children or young adults have had radiation therapy to the chest area as treatment for another cancer (such as Hodgkin's disease or non-Hodgkin's lymphoma) are at significantly increased risk for breast cancer. Some reports found the risk to be twelve times the normal risk. This varies with the age of the patient at the time of radiation. Younger patients have a higher risk. If chemotherapy was also given, the risk may be lowered if the chemotherapy stops ovarian hormone production.

Women in this situation should discuss this risk with their GP or the oncologist who originally treated them, and may want to pursue preventative measures similar to those taken by women with hereditary breast cancer risk.

Reproductive History

The following factors related to your reproductive history can increase risk, but the increase is small:

- Having your first period before age twelve
- Having no children
- Having your first child after age thirty
- Starting menopause after age fifty-five
- Taking hormone replacement therapy (HRT) for symptoms of menopause

Age at the Start of Your First Period　　Girls who start menstruating before age twelve appear to be at higher risk for breast cancer than those who start later. The reason could be that hormones, such as estrogen, which are increased when a girl begins having periods, contribute to developing breast cancer. The longer a woman has periods, the greater her exposure to estrogen.

Age at the Start of Your Menopause　　Women who begin menopause later than average (older than fifty to fifty-two), are at a higher risk for breast cancer than women who start earlier. Again, the reason might be that the later menopause begins, the longer a woman is exposed to increased hormone levels associated with having her regular periods. Women who have menopause surgically induced by removal of the uterus might still have a higher risk if their ovaries are still producing estrogen.

Risk Factors Related to Lifestyle and Personal Choices

Age at the Birth of Your First Child　　Women who have never delivered a child are at higher risk for breast cancer than those who have. Women who have had a first birth after age thirty are at greater risk than women who have had children before thirty. The reason may be that an early pregnancy causes protective changes in the breast tissue, causing the breast cell to mature in some way that differs from the changes that occur later in life.

Hormone Replacement Therapy (HRT)　　Hormone replacement therapy (HRT) refers to treatment with pills or skin patches that contain estrogen or estrogen and progesterone combined. Hormones are chemicals that affect the activity of certain cells and organs. Both estrogen and progesterone play an important role in a woman's life, regulating menstrual periods and affecting the growth of breast tissue. The ovaries produce these particular hormones, but they can also be made in a laboratory or obtained from plants and animals.

As women leave their childbearing years behind, they begin to produce less estrogen and progesterone. A lack of estrogen can lead to unpleasant menopausal symptoms, such as hot flashes and vaginal dryness. It can also contribute to osteoporosis—the loss of bone tissue. HRT is often prescribed to relieve menopausal symptoms and was thought to reduce the risk of osteoporosis. HRT may also be prescribed when a woman experiences premature menopause, whether naturally or as the result of medical treatment. Recent findings about the benefits of HRT suggest it be used cautiously and for shorter duration. HRT is associated with a twofold increase in breast cancer risk.

If you are having problems with menopausal symptoms and are thinking about taking herbal supplements to relieve the discomfort of mood swings, vaginal dryness, night sweats, or other problems, discuss this first with a pharmacist. Some herbal supplements contain natural-source estrogens—but these are still estrogens and can affect breast cancer risk and recurrence the same as other forms of hormone replacement therapy.

Obesity   Being 40 percent above the ideal body weight greatly increases a person's risk of certain types of cancers. Because estrogen—a hormone that has been linked to breast cancer development—is stored in fatty or "adipose" tissue, the more fat we have, the more estrogen is available to influence our endocrine systems and breast tissue.

The extent to which a woman is overweight at the time of her diagnosis may influence the chance of getting breast cancer again. Many women consider a healthy diet and exercise an important part of healing, recovery, and maintaining well-being.

WHAT IS BREAST CANCER?

Diet/Nutrition   The total number of calories and the amount of fat you eat on a regular basis might influence your risk for breast cancer. However, there has not been extensive research on individual women to prove this. More and more we hear of the importance of eating a varied and well-balanced diet, emphasizing fruits and vegetables, low-fat, high-fiber foods, and increasing physical activity. In addition, some researchers have found that certain vitamins (such as A, C, and E) and selenium, which are also known as antioxidants, might help to prevent cancer.

Factors of Uncertain, Controversial, or Unproven Effect on Breast Cancer Risk

Antiperspirants: Internet e-mail rumors have suggested that chemicals in underarm antiperspirants are absorbed through the skin, interfere with lymph circulation, and cause toxins to build up in the breast, and eventually lead to breast cancer. There is very little experimental or epidemiological (studies of the causes and transmission of diseases) evidence to support this rumor. Chemicals in products, such as antiperspirants, are tested thoroughly to ensure their safety. One small study recently found trace levels of parabens (used as preservatives in antiperspirants), which have weak estrogen-like properties, in a small sample of breast cancer tumors. However, the study did not look at whether parabens caused the tumors. This was a preliminary finding, and more research is needed to determine what effect, if any, parabens might have on breast cancer risk. On the other hand, a recent large epidemiological study found no increase in breast cancer in women who used underarm antiperspirants or shaved their underarms.

Underwire bras: Internet e-mail rumors and at least one book have suggested that bras cause breast cancer by obstructing lymph flow. There is no scientific or clinical basis for that claim.

Induced abortion: Several studies have provided very strong data that induced abortions have no overall effect on the risk of breast cancer. Also, there is no evidence of a direct relationship between breast cancer and spontaneous abortion (miscarriage) in most of the studies that have been published. Scientists invited to participate in a conference on abortion and breast cancer by the U.S. National Cancer Institute (February 2003) concluded that there was no relationship. A recent report of 83,000 women with breast cancer found no link to a previous abortion, either spontaneous (stillbirth) or induced.

Breast implants: Several studies have found that breast implants do not increase breast cancer risk, although silicone breast implants can cause scar tissue to form in the breast. Implants make it harder to see breast tissue on standard mammograms, but additional X-ray pictures— called implant displacement views—can be used to examine the breast tissue more thoroughly.

Environmental pollution: A great deal of research has been reported and more is being done to understand environmental influences on breast cancer risk. The goal is to determine their possible relationships to breast cancer.

Currently, research does not show a clear link between breast cancer risk and exposure to environmental pollutants, such as the pesticide DDE (chemically related to dichloro-diphenyl-trichloroethane, or DDT), and PCBS (polychlorinated biphenyls).

Smoking: Most studies have found no link between active cigarette smoking and breast cancer. Though both active smoking and second-hand smoke have been suggested to increase the risk of breast cancer in some studies, the issue remains controversial. The California Environmental Protection Agency recently concluded that second-hand smoke causes breast cancer in younger, mainly premenopausal women. The U.S. Surgeon General is currently reviewing the evidence on this link, and a report is expected in late 2006. Regardless of the possible link between tobacco and breast cancer, not smoking ciga-rettes and limiting exposure to secondhand smoke is beneficial for a number of health reasons, including a reduced risk of other cancers and heart disease.

Night work: A few recent studies have suggested that women who work at night—for example, nurses on a night shift—have an increased risk of developing breast cancer. However, this increased risk has not yet been proven, and when further studies are conducted, this factor may be found to be unimportant.

Birth Control Pills

The hormones that our bodies produce play a role in the development of breast cancer. This is why the age at which we start menstruating, have (or don't have) children, and go through menopause can all influ-ence whether we are at risk. Increasingly, researchers are also focusing on the relationship between breast cancer and other hormones, including those to which we are exposed in the environment and those that we might take in the form of birth control pills. Some studies show that taking birth control pills for more than five years could put us at a higher risk for breast cancer, while others indicate no link. The research is far from conclusive.

MINIMIZING YOUR RISK

While there are risk factors for breast cancer that you cannot change (such as age, family history, or reproductive history), you can substantially reduce your risk by making positive changes to your lifestyle.

+ Lose excess weight. Even a small degree of excess weight, 5 kg (11 lbs. and greater) is associated with increased breast cancer risk, especially among postmenopausal women.
+ Be physically active. Studies show that even moderate physical activity can reduce your risk by 30 to 40 percent. Choose an exercise or activity that makes you feel warm and breathe harder (such as brisk walking) for at least thirty minutes on five or more days of the week.
+ Limit your intake of alcohol. Women who drink alcohol have a modestly increased risk. The more you drink, the greater your risk. Limit yourself to not more than one drink per day—12 ounces (340 mL) of beer, 5 ounces (140 mL) of wine, or 1.5 ounces (42 mL) of spirits.
+ Breastfeed your baby if you are able. Breast-feeding seems to offer some women protection against breast cancer and it's good for the baby. If you can, breastfeed for at least four months.
+ Quit smoking. Smoking tobacco and breathing secondhand smoke have been linked in some studies to breast cancer. Tobacco smoke is responsible for 30 percent of all cancer deaths.
+ Talk to your doctor about the risks and benefits of hormone replacement therapy (HRT). HRT can relieve symptoms of menopause and reduces the risk of osteoporosis and colon cancer.

WHAT IS BREAST CANCER?

However, HRT increases the risk of breast cancer and heart disease.

♦ Although there is no compelling evidence suggesting that exposure to pesticides and other potentially harmful chemicals is related to breast cancer risk, it would still be prudent to minimize exposure to these agents. Follow the warnings and handling procedures in material safety data sheets (MSDSS), which are available for most chemicals. Work with your employer to ensure that your workplace has good air quality and that chemicals are properly handled.

SUMMARY

It appears that breast cells may be very sensitive to radiation, diet, hormonal changes, pregnancy, and environmental toxins during adolescence and the early teen years. This sensitivity may result in cellular changes, which can increase or decrease the likelihood of developing breast cancer later in life. Today, we don't have much control over these factors.

Finding out you have cancer is one of the most difficult experiences you will go through. Many women say the first months were the worst: making decisions about things they didn't really understand at first, telling family and friends about the diagnosis, adjusting to new doctors, hospitals, and treatment centers, and feeling "out of control."

Waiting several days before making treatment decisions, or starting treatment, to find out what you need to know will not change what will happen to you. Allowing yourself the time to consider different options, to talk to surgeons and oncologists, and to talk to other women who have had breast cancer is a reasonable thing for you to do in this confusing and frightening period. Take the time you need to feel ready for the next step, but don't wait around hoping to hear what you want to hear.

No one knows for certain why some people get cancer, while others who live the same lifestyle or inherit the same genes don't get it. Dr. Susan Love, a leading U.S. breast cancer expert and advocate, has written, "People have the tendency to blame themselves for being ill... You didn't create your own cancer by eating too much sugar or thinking negative thoughts or allowing yourself to be too stressed out."

WHAT IS BREAST CANCER?

No one can tell you exactly what happened to cause you to develop breast cancer. But you do have control over your treatment choices and what you do to help yourself to become well again.

There's a universal myth of the hero who travels to the underworld, endures hardship and returns to her people with hard-won wisdom. That's the story we hear from the women who come through their cancer treatment with their eyes wide open.

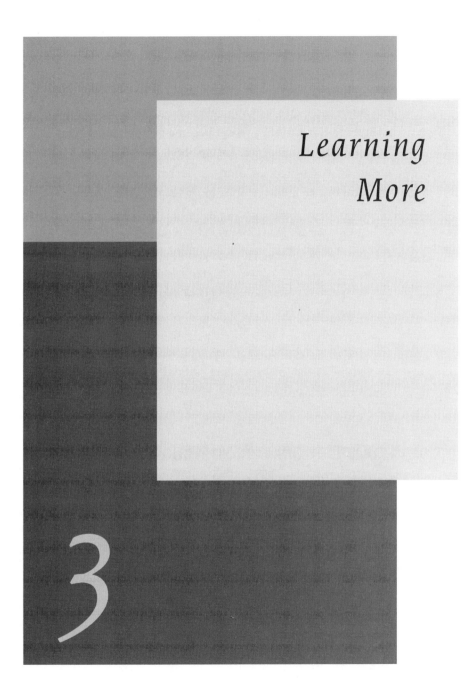

Learning More

3

A generation ago, most of the diagnostic tests used to monitor cancer did not exist. Nor did the range of treatment options. Although the push has been for patients to be more knowledgeable about their care, as you read through the mountains of unfiltered information, you can become overwhelmed. This chapter explains basic information about diagnostic tests, characteristics, and prognosis, along with the different types of breast cancer, to help you start to understand the disease.

Cancer is not who I am; it's what I had. I am not a victim; I am an overcomer. Just like I had a car accident two years ago and got over it, I had cancer. I don't think about it every day. I didn't and don't want special treatment, but I did covet the learning, the help, the advice, and the prayers.

The doctors are trying to map out exactly what is wrong with you and they're giving it to you in sophisticated medical terms. It's like being in a foreign county: you don't speak the language, and you're trying to find directions.

What Can My Doctor Tell Me about My Breast Cancer?

The first step in deciding which treatment is right for you is to understand as much as you can about *your* tumor. The following tests are commonly used after a surgeon has removed the suspicious or cancerous lump from your breast, in order to diagnose your cancer, determine the extent of the disease, and help you understand which treatments are right for your type of cancer.

BIOPSY

When your cancer was diagnosed, some tissue was removed from your breast so it could be analyzed. This is called a "biopsy." This procedure might have been done with a syringe that is inserted into the lump, drawing a small amount of fluid with suction (a process called "cytology aspirate" or "fine-needle aspiration biopsy"). If the lump is suspected to be a cyst (a small harmless sac of fluid), an ultrasound exam or fine needle aspiration (FNA) can help confirm it. If the fluid drawn out by the FNA is bloody, it will be sent for testing. If it is not, the lump is just a cyst and no further testing need be done. The lump will go away once the fluid is removed.

Other kinds of biopsies include inserting a long needle into the side of the lump (a "core biopsy" or "incisional biopsy") or cutting out the lump through surgery ("excisional biopsy"). Although fine needle biopsy can be useful, the current standard of care, and the most common initial procedure, is the core biopsy to diagnose the tumor. Material from a core biopsy—unlike FNA—can provide additional information for testing.

A pathologist will examine the removed tissue and write a report about what was found. Details about the tumor's appearance help provide information about the type of breast cancer. This information will be helpful in planning your treatment. The pathologist also examines and describes the features of the cancer in detail so that a prognosis— the likely course and outcome of a disease and/or treatments for the disease—can be made.

Although your surgeon might be able to remove the entire mass of tumor from your breast at the time of your biopsy, this is just the first step in your treatment plan. Should the results of your biopsy indicate the need for a lumpectomy or mastectomy, there are advantages for you in having the same surgeon perform both the biopsy and any subsequent surgery as s/he can position the breast and plan the surgery to minimize scarring. The biopsy tissue removed from your breast will be sent to the pathology lab for careful study and testing to determine how the cancer is likely to behave in the future and what treatment options work best.

> *I think the hardest times for me were waiting for lab results—I knew I had cancer but I didn't know how much cancer I had. Just waiting and hoping to hear the news seemed the hardest part of the treatments.*

AXILLARY LYMPH NODES

After you have had the surgery to remove the cancerous lump, the pathologist will examine the breast tissue and the lymph nodes that were removed from the armpit area. There are approximately twenty-five to sixty lymph nodes under each arm, and some of these will have been removed at the time of your surgery and examined under the microscope. At least ten nodes should be examined. If the nodes contain cancer cells (this is called being "node-positive"), it is likely that cancer cells have spread to other parts of the body. The number of lymph nodes, if any, involved with the tumor is one of the most important factors in determining a prognosis.

THE PATHOLOGY REPORT

The pathology report should indicate whether or not the cancer cells are spreading. Cancer that is spreading, also known as "invasive cancer" or "infiltrating cancer," has grown outside the basement membrane of the cells and into the surrounding tissue. This is different from a condition known as "carcinoma in situ," which is not cancerous but can indicate that cancer could develop. There are other factors that should be described in the report. They indicate the seriousness of the disease:

- The number (if any) of lymph nodes involved

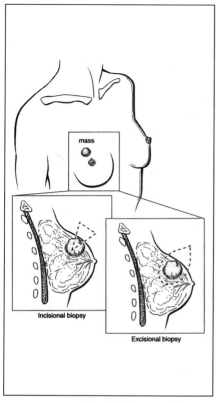

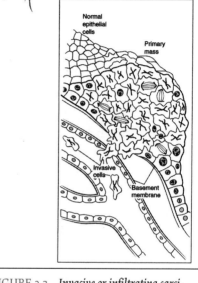

FIGURE 3.1   *Incisional and excisional biopsy*

FIGURE 3.2   *Invasive or infiltrating carcinoma, showing that the tumor has broken through the basement membrane and cells are shed into the blood and lymph system*

- The size of the tumor at the time of diagnosis
- The grade of the tumor (grade means whether the cells are aggressive or benign looking)
- The extent to which the cancer cells are spreading into the surrounding tissue (called margins)
- The presence of tumor cells in blood or lymph vessels
- The hormone receptor status (whether the tumor is highly sensitive to the influence of hormones)

- The HER2/neu status (whether the tumor expresses HER2/neu oncogene)

Tumor Size

The size of the tumor predicts for recurrence. If the tumor is less than 1 cm, there is a low chance of it returning. On the other hand, if it is 3 cm or more it is considered large and there is a higher chance of recurrence.

Histologic Grade

Once the pathologist has determined what kind of breast cancer you have, s/he will then look more closely at the characteristics and "activity" of the tumor cells. To classify the grade of the breast cancer cell the pathologist will look at the nucleus of the cell (the central organelle that contains the cell's DNA and its controlling mechanisms), cell division (called mitosis), and the tubule formation (percentage of the cancer composed of tubular structures).

TABLE 2: FEATURES OF THE PATHOLOGY REPORT

THE TUMOR:

Size: measured in centimeters

Type: in situ, invasive, or mixed

Invasion: Lymphovascular invasion: presence or absence of tumor cells in the lymphatic tissues (called lymphovascular invasion) or vascular spaces

Grade: I, II, or III

Number of mitotic divisions: rate of growth

Necrosis if DCIS

Surgical resection margins: presence or absence of tumor

THE LYMPH NODES:

Total number of lymph nodes removed

Number of nodes with cancer

Size of nodes

Extra-nodal extension—growth beyond the walls of the lymph nodes

Sentinel node biopsy: performed or not

THE TUMOR:

ER and PR status: positive or negative receptors for estrogen or
  progesterone

HER2/neu status: positive or
  negative

Resection margins: free, involved,
  or close, and if close, how
  close?

These features are closely examined to determine a cancer's grade: nuclear grade, mitotic grade, and tubular grade. Each of these features is measured on a scale of 1 to 3, with 1 being the least aggressive and 3 being the most aggressive. The scores of each of the cell's features are then added together for a final sum that will range from 3 to 9.

- *Nuclear grade* refers to the change in shape of the cells. They sometimes refer to the tumors as being "wild-looking" or poorly differentiated, meaning the tumor growth is very active and the cancer cells look very different from normal breast cells. Odd-shaped, wild-looking, or unusual-looking cells are thought to be more aggressive. Cells that look closer to normal are usually less aggressive.
- *Mitotic grade* refers to how many and how quickly cells are dividing. The most aggressive cancers tend to have many cells dividing at the same time, growing more rapidly. Less aggressive cancers tend to have very few dividing cells.
- *Tubular grade* (or the percentage of cancer composed of tubular structures) is the third indicator. Less aggressive cancers have less than 10 percent, and more aggressive cancers have more than 75 percent.

Lymphovascular Invasion

The pathologist will also look to see if there are any cancer cells in the middle of the blood vessels or lymph vessels in the breast tissue. When cancer cells are found here, the cancer is also in the lymph system.

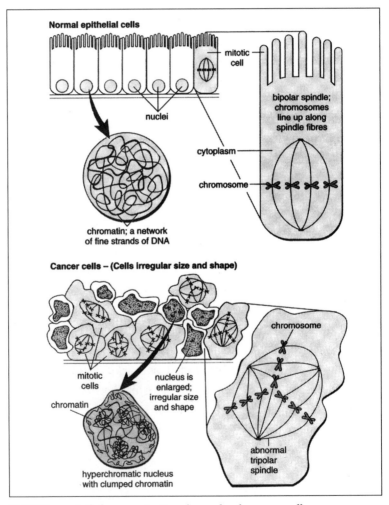

FIGURE 3.3   *Pathology examination of normal and cancerous cells*

Estrogen Receptor Test and Progesterone Receptor Test

Pathologists perform other tests on the tissue or tumor that was removed from your breast. The tests conducted will vary depending on your hospital. Two tests that determine whether the tumor is sensitive to certain hormones are the estrogen receptor (ER) test and the progesterone receptor (PR) test. If the tumors are found to be sensitive to these hormones, we say they are estrogen receptor positive or progesterone receptor positive. The tumors have binding or docking sites on the surface of their cells where the hormone proteins can attach and cause changes in the cell growth.

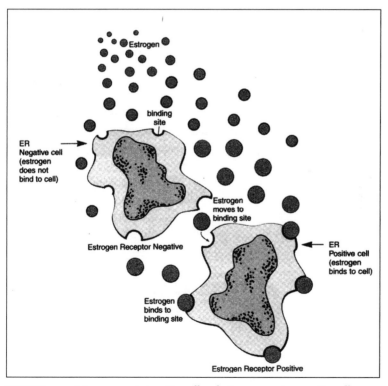

FIGURE 3.4   *Estrogen receptor positive cell and estrogen receptor negative cell*

Usually, women who have already been through menopause are estrogen receptor positive and those who have not are estrogen receptor negative; but this isn't always true, so the tests are important. Tumors that are ER positive can often be successfully treated with anti-estrogen drugs, such as tamoxifen or aromatase inhibitors. ER positive tumors are generally slower growing than ER negative tumors.

HER2/NEU ONCOGENE

Measurement of HER2/neu oncogene has recently emerged as a very important factor. Oncogenes are genes that lead to cancer or cancer growth. About 25 percent of breast cancer patients appear to have overexpression or amplification of the HER2/neu (human epidermal growth factor receptor 2) oncogene, which leads to the production of a great deal of protein—this is called overexpression. The oncogene contains the code that makes an important protein in the cancer cell, tyrosine kinase. This gene is often associated with a more active or aggressive disease and a worse prognosis. A new drug called trastuzumab (Herceptin) acts against tumors that overexpress HER2/neu. The gene tests to determine the presence of HER2/neu are performed on a portion of the biopsy specimen.

There are two methods used to perform this test. The first, and most common, is called immunohistochemistry. If the results of this test are not clear-cut, then the fluorescent in situ hybridization test (FISH) will be done.

FLOW CYTOMETRY AND S-PHASE FRACTION
ACTIVITY TESTS

Other tests that are sometimes used to measure the activity level of tumor cells are the flow cytometry test and the S-phase fraction activity test. Breast cancer's "S-phase fraction" (SPF) is the percentage of cancer cells replicating their DNA. DNA replication usually signals that a

74

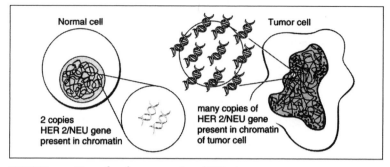

FIGURE 3.5   *Normal and overexpression of HER-2/neu oncogene*

cell is getting ready to split into two new cells. A low SPF indicates the cancer is growing fairly slowly and a high SPF shows the cell is growing rapidly. Rapidly growing tumors need to be treated with more aggressive treatments than those that grow slowly.

Whether these tests add any significant new information, compared to older tests in predicting how a woman's breast cancer develops, is questionable. Although these tests were once very common, they are no longer routinely done in the United States or Canada.

Gene Profiling/Expression Mapping

In the last few years, new techniques have become available to map certain gene profiles that are particular to breast cancer. These patterns of gene expression can be used to classify the tumors into different groups based on the likelihood of either a good outcome or a poor prognosis. The tests for gene profiling are currently being assessed for the usefulness of the information they provide. Currently, we don't know if these expensive new tests add anything more than the standard battery of tests.

One improvement that needs to be made is the waiting time between tests and diagnosis. It is hard to feel optimistic when you don't know what you're facing.

Once your breast cancer tumor has been studied and a pathology report made, imaging and other tests may be done to determine if the cancer has spread beyond your breast. Some of these tests may be done by your family doctor or surgeon, and other tests may be requested by your oncologist.

There are also good reasons for not doing these tests. They are expensive, and the chance of finding anything is relatively low. Again, remember that you have some choice in whether you want these tests. Ask your doctor what new information they might provide and how they will affect your treatment. Usually, it will take between two and seven days to receive the results of the biopsy and pathology tests. Scan results can take longer.

Tests That May Be Used to Determine if Cancer Has Spread

BONE SCANS

This test is an imaging method that indicates if the cancer has spread to bone tissue. To get the image of the inside of the bone, a small amount of radioactive dye is injected into a vein, which is then carried throughout your system. In places where there is a cancerous tumor, the radioactive dye will accumulate and the image will indicate that an abnormality is present.

At fifty-seven, it's a little late to be starting medical school. But the burden still falls on me, having to pick among options.

COMPUTERIZED AXIAL TOMOGRAPHY (CAT) SCANS

In this test, a computer takes multiple X-rays from many different angles and combines them to create a cross-sectional picture of the internal organs. CAT scans are painless and are usually performed in the X-ray department of hospitals. They can detect the spread of disease to internal organs.

MAGNETIC RESONANCE IMAGING (MRI) SCANS

Another painless method of imaging is the MRI. MRI scans use radio waves and magnets that are painlessly directed through your body to produce detailed images of internal organs.

POSITRON EMISSION TOMOGRAPHY (PET) SCANS

A PET scan is a procedure in which a small amount of radioactive glucose (sugar) is injected into a vein, and a scanner is used to make detailed, computerized pictures of areas inside the body where the glucose is used. Because cancer cells often use more glucose than normal cells, the pictures can be used to find cancer cells in the body.

How Can I Know What Stage My Cancer Is At?

Staging is the process of finding out how much cancer there is in your body and where it is located. Knowing the stage of your cancer will help your doctor determine your prognosis and suggest the most effective treatments for you. Staging is determined by:

- the size of your tumor
- whether lymph nodes are involved and, if so, how many
- indications of metastasis or spread of the cancer cells beyond the breast tissue at the time of prognosis

You might hear your cancer classified using the TNM Classification System. The stage of your cancer is directly related to the possibility of it spreading and causing future problems.

Tumors are designated the letter T (tumor size), N (palpable nodes or nodes that can be felt by physical exam), and/or M (metastasis or spread of cancer beyond the breast tissue to distant organs or bones).

The stage of breast cancer describes its size and the extent to which it has spread. The staging system ranges from Stage I to Stage IV.

STAGE	TUMOR SIZE	LYMPH NODE INVOLVEMENT	METASTASIS (SPREAD)
I	less than 2 cm	No	No
II	between 2–5 cm	No, or in same side	No
III	more than 5 cm	Yes, on same side	No
IV	not applicable	Not applicable	Yes

When most cancers are found, they are at the stage I or stage II levels. At these stages they are highly treatable—more than 90 percent of women whose cancers are diagnosed at stage I or stage II levels are alive five years later. Your doctor determines the stage by asking questions (taking a history), performing a physical examination, and doing additional tests.

In practice, oncologists often stage the tumor before ordering additional tests. Tests that can help determine the extent of your cancer include chest X-rays, bone scans, and blood tests that determine how your liver is functioning. Chest X-rays and mammograms are part of your initial assessment, and mammograms will continue to be done in the years following your treatment. Computerized axial tomography (CAT) scans and magnetic resonance imaging (MRI) scans are sometimes used if more information is needed or if the other tests don't provide enough information.

BREAST CANCER SURVIVAL BY STAGE

The numbers below are based on patients diagnosed from 1995 to 1998 and can be expected to be a little different for women diagnosed more recently. One reason is that the staging system was revised in 2002. Another reason is that treatments have improved since 1998. Because of these improved treatments, the survival rates for women diagnosed now should be better. These numbers come from the American College of Surgeons National Cancer Data Base.

STAGE	FIVE-YEAR RELATIVE SURVIVAL RATE
0	100%
I	100%
IIA	92%
IIB	81%
IIIA	67%
IIIB	54%
IV	20%

The five-year survival rate refers to the percentage of patients who live at least five years after their cancer is diagnosed. Five-year rates are used to produce a standard way of discussing prognosis. Of course, many people live much longer than five years. Five-year relative survival rates assume that people will die of other causes and compares the observed survival with that expected for people without breast cancer. That means that relative survival only talks about deaths from breast cancer.

> *I just can't go into my treatment ignorant, although in a way I am. I would just feel like I wasn't doing my part.*

Doctors and patients feel the benefits and the burdens of medical information being so accessible to patients. Yet studies show that the more informed patients are about their care, the more they feel in control of their emotions and the more likely their health will improve. Additionally, patients who feel knowledgeable and informed about their disease and treatments are often more hopeful, and they maintain self-confidence and are better able to communicate with their health care team.

> *The patients are stressed, they're so confused and it's in our laps. They are deserving of guidance and compassion.*

SUMMARY

Cancer information is complex, confusing, and ever changing. You might be feeling overwhelmed with the emotional aspects of a cancer diagnosis. The information might be hard to understand. It's okay to ask questions even months or years after your diagnosis. Your doctor won't think less of you and won't consider your questions stupid or repetitive. S/he is a professional whose job is to be helpful and kind to you—not to judge you. *You* decide when you need the information.

The pathology report and other tests and scans will provide you with information that you and your doctor can use to make decisions about what to do next. Although it is only natural to assume that "more is better" when it comes to tests, you should ask your doctor to explain the tests and procedures so that you can make an informed decision about which might be useful. It is also important to remember that some newer tests do not give any more information than the traditional markers of cancer (size, grade, hormone receptor status, and involvement of the lymph nodes), which have been used for a long time.

Staging your cancer will give you, and your doctors, information to plan the best treatments, help doctors communicate with each other about your case, and help to anticipate the course your disease is likely to take.

The information is based on studying many thousands of people with cancer. Although no one can predict exactly what will happen to you, it is important to understand the amount of cancer in your body in order to plan appropriate care.

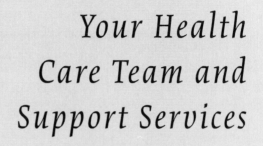

*Your Health
Care Team and
Support Services*

4

This chapter is a guide to some of the people—health care professionals and others—who can help you through diagnosis and treatment. You will also find questions that you might want to ask the people who are helping along the way.

The care and concern shown me has been unbelievable. It is a refreshing change to be treated as a human being dealing with a horrendous disease instead of just another number.

I believe a few kind words from the doctor can go a long way.

The Other "Big C"—Communication!

Before we talk about the people who are available to help you through diagnosis and treatment, let's have a word about communication and decision-making styles. Some women are comfortable knowing very little information about their own cancer diagnosis and prefer to leave the decision making to someone else, such as a doctor they know and trust. Others want to actively participate in their diagnosis and treatment and may choose to discuss their treatment plan with family members before making any decisions. These women often feel more in control when they have this information explained to them in a way that they can understand.

I did research for two or three weeks…I went to fifteen or twenty Web sites because I needed to know everything they were going to do to me. But the Web was messing me up: I got confused because I didn't understand it. I really needed to do this but I needed advice from my nurse to make my decisions.

No matter what your decision-making style, if you change your mind and want to talk more or less, or if you decide you want more or less information or more or less involvement in the decision making, tell your doctor. Doctors and nurses are often very good at understanding human behavior or sensing discomfort, but no one can read your mind. You'll also save yourself some time if you can make clear and understandable requests.

> I didn't know if the doctor was going to be the cheerleader and advisor that I was longing for. So my gatekeeper is my friend, not my doctor. We hash it all out, and we figure the options. She has a good, clear, focused head about all this stuff... and she has a great sense of humor about it all.

Try to prepare for your cancer appointments with your clinic or doctor just as you would for other important meetings. You might choose to ask a family member or a trusted friend to accompany you to the appointments and help you decide what to do or act as a sounding board. Try keeping a small notebook with you to write down questions, appointment times, the names of the drugs, and the phone numbers of new people you will meet. Cancer questions or concerns can come up at any time, and some treatments cause you to become weary or forgetful. The notebook can become a useful tool or journal for your many thoughts and questions during therapy. Here are some other hints and tips:

- Plan ahead for doctor's appointments and keep a written record of questions and concerns.
- Bring a friend or family member whose job is to help remember what is said during the appointment.

- Bring paper and pen or a tape recorder. Let the doctor know if you want to record the meeting.
- Call ahead and ask how much time you will have for your first appointment. Let the office know if you will need a longer time or another appointment.
- Ask about directions and parking, then you won't worry about them when it's time for your appointment.
- Bring along any medications, vitamins, or other treatments you are taking. It won't help if you say you take "half a green pill and one red tablet."
- Tell your doctor about any other treatments or therapies such as acupuncture, herbs, vitamins, visualization, or spiritual practice that you consider important to healing.

When You Get Home

1. **Review the visit.** To help you to remember clearly what you and your doctor talked about, review the notes from the visit.
2. **Keep a journal.** Make a note of your visits, names, phone numbers, contact information, symptoms, prescribed medications, reactions to treatment, and questions as they occur. Write down your thoughts, encouraging words, expectations. Read them over before your next visit.
3. **Learn some basic medical terms.** This will help you understand and follow your progress, feel more in control, and help manage your care.
4. **Get more information if you need it.** If you are worried about your progress, your test results, or the treatment options the doctors (in all likelihood you will have more than one doctor responsible for your care) have given you, find out more before

making a decision. Discuss your concerns with your family doctor and, if you would feel more reassured, ask for a second opinion. Then, when you've had time to think, make another appointment with the original doctor or specialist.

Remember that the people who are going to care for you during cancer treatments are on your side and they know this is a very difficult time for you and your family. They are there to help you and make the treatments as understandable as possible. *You* are the most important person on your cancer care team. *You* are the person who must make the decisions about your own care, based on the best possible advice.

Making decisions about your treatment and understanding what will happen to you might already be difficult. If you feel more comfortable speaking in a language other than English, you will probably find it helpful to bring along a friend or family member or someone from your community who can help you.

Again, only you can determine how much information you are comfortable absorbing. It will be different for each woman. If you want this information, and when you are ready to hear it, ask your doctor to write down the name of your type of breast cancer, the size of your tumor, your test results, and stage of the disease.

> *I will let the doctors treat me but the rest is up to me—whether it is mental change, cleansing teas, or exercise. Maybe by working together I will live longer or we will find a cure. I am living with cancer, not dying with cancer.*

You may have to ask more than once to be sure you understand your treatments. As mentioned earlier, cancer information is complex and ever changing. You have the right to be given clear answers to your questions. Keep asking questions until you know everything that you want and need to know.

Who Can Help Me Get Through All This?

"Is there anything I can do?" "What do you need?" Over and over, that's what I heard from friends when I had a return of breast cancer.

I had surgery, eight chemotherapy sessions, then five weeks of radiation ahead of me. Seven and a half months of treatment that would begin in a July heat wave and end in the last dreary days of February.

I knew my friends cared about me. I'm a widow, I live alone and I would turn seventy in the middle of the treatments. Of course they wanted to help. What my friends didn't understand was how hard it was to respond to those questions, partly because I didn't know what I needed, but also because I was hesitant to tell them what I did need.

But I did need help, and, of course, my kind and clever friends soon figured out what they could do.

—BERYL YOUNG

YOUR FAMILY DOCTOR

Your family doctor is probably the first person you will consult. S/he will remain an important part of your cancer care team. Family physicians rarely treat cancer but they can and do refer you to specialists. Your family doctor can be there to answer questions, and can play an important role in coordination, consultation, and communication. S/he can be your advocate in the hospital or treatment center. Ask your family doctor to refer you to a specialist in breast changes and breast cancer. Your ability to choose will depend on whether you live in or near a large urban center. If you aren't comfortable going to your appointments alone, or don't want to ask the questions yourself, ask a close friend, family member, or a woman who has been through what you are going through to help you out.

> *I was just a teacher but I had to do something for my sister to deal with all my nervous energy. Like a lot of people, I was feeling frightened and help-less and didn't know what to say. So I turned into a Googling machine. Doing the homework gave me the comforting illusion of being "in control."*

Find a family doctor you are comfortable with if you do not already have one. Some women prefer an old-fashioned, protective physician who tells them what they feel is best for them. Other women like to know all about their illness in order to feel more in control. There is no right or wrong approach to this relationship. Like all long-term rela-tionships, it is important to trust, communicate, and respect one another. This might be a lifelong relationship and requires effort by both you and your doctor.

If there is a shortage of family doctors in the area where you live, you might want to review the section in this book "If You Have a Problem Talking with Your Doctor." In other words, if you can't find a doctor you like, consider exploring how to work with the one you have.

> *Few patients realize how deeply they can affect their doctors. That is a big secret in medicine. We think about, talk about, dream about our patients. We went into clinical medicine because we like dealing on a personal level with people who have chosen to put their bodies in our*

hands. Our patients make or break our days. Massaging the ego is key to manipulating responsible people like doctors. When we feel your trust, you have us.

You might also want to ask your family doctor whether you should be referred to an oncologist (cancer specialist) before surgery, if this is an option where you live. Sometimes the oncologist will consult with you and the surgeon about a treatment plan before surgery.

Doctors must look at the patient as a whole person. Patients must inform their physicians about what they expect from their health care providers. But God bless you if you do that. I wish people would realize that the fighters are also the survivors—they are fighting for their lives.

YOUR SURGEON

In most hospitals, there are different types of surgeons, some of whom specialize in breast surgery. If there is such a specialist in your hospital, this is likely whom you will see. There are some questions that you might want to ask your surgeon (or surgeons):

♦ How many breast cancer patients do you treat each year?
♦ Do you have a preference for a certain type of surgical treatment?
♦ What treatment do you recommend for me and why?
♦ Are there advantages for me if my surgery is done at a particular time in my menstrual cycle (if you are still menstruating)?
♦ Can you put me in touch with a local breast cancer support group?
♦ Can you tell me what my options are for breast reconstruction? (This does not mean you have to choose a breast reconstruction— just that you want the information.)
♦ Can you show me a photo of what my breast might look like after surgery?

♦ Can I speak with another woman you have treated?

You might want to take your husband, friend, partner, son, or daughter for support. Write down your questions and the answers. If it is difficult for you to take notes, consider taping the conversation, but let your doctor know beforehand.

Many cancer support groups have peer visitor programs for women with breast cancer. Breast cancer survivors are trained to provide support to women going through the experience of breast cancer. They can do this in the hospital, at home, or over the telephone, and are matched as closely as possible by age, type of surgery, and treatment. They provide support and a free information kit, which includes booklets and other useful items.

> I found my cancer center the most caring and professional one you could wish for. One treatment nurse said to me, "You are now a cancer patient—you belong to us. We will care for you both now and after treatment and for periodic checkups afterward by your oncologist." These people are the greatest.

YOUR ONCOLOGIST

Again, depending on whether or not you live in or near a large urban center, you could be referred to an oncologist. This is the doctor whose training and experience deal particularly with cancer. Some oncologists deal with specific types of cancer (e.g., breast, brain, or lung). The two main types of oncologists are "medical oncologists" and "radiation oncologists." Medical oncologists provide systemic therapies, including chemotherapy. Radiation oncologists provide radiation treatments. Both types of treatment can be given after surgery to prevent cancer from returning.

Even if you do not have treatment after surgery, you may want to speak to an oncologist or even have your follow-up care with an oncologist. Follow-up care is the care you will need following your surgery. For some women an oncologist may not be necessary or, in certain regions of the country, available. In this case, you should see your family doctor for follow-up care.

These are some questions you or someone close to you may want to ask your oncologist or family doctor:

- What type of breast cancer do I have and at what stage is the disease?
- What treatments are you recommending for me and why?
- How will the treatments help me?
- What are the risks of the treatments?
- What can I expect to happen to me if I choose *not* to have these treatments?
- Will the treatments be painful? If so, how can the pain be managed?
- When and where will the treatments take place?
- What are the usual side effects? What can you recommend to reduce the side effects?
- How long can I expect the treatments to take?
- If I miss a treatment, can I make it up?
- What problems should I report to you?
- How can I contact you between visits?
- Can I take other medication during treatments?
- Is there anything I shouldn't eat or drink during these treatments, such as alcohol?
- What's the longest I can wait before having these treatments? (Some women want more time to fully recover from the surgery.)
- Can you put me in touch with a local breast cancer support group?
- If we get rid of the cancer, what are the chances of it coming back?

Young women, for whom having children is a priority, might want to ask the following questions as well. It is important to ask these questions before you embark on a treatment path because both chemotherapy and radiation can have serious and permanent implications for your ability to have children.

- Will my treatments affect my reproductive system and my ability to have children?
- Are there alternative ways to treat my cancer without damaging my reproductive system?
- Can I preserve my eggs so that I can try to get pregnant after treatment?
- How will I know if my reproductive system was affected and/or damaged once my treatments are over?

In addition, fertility issues are addressed by the American Society for Clinical Oncology in the recently released Fertility Preservation Clinical Practice Guideline.

The Clinical Practice Guideline "ASCO Recommendations on Fertility Preservation in People Treated for Cancer" is now available online at www.asco.org. The guideline was developed by the ASCO Fertility Preservation Expert Panel, which recommends that any oncologist discussing cancer therapy with reproductive-age patients address potential treatment-related infertility with them or, in the case of children, with their parents.

> *Following my diagnosis and lumpectomy I felt fear every time I thought about the cancer. I bought a new car because my old one was rusting and I associated rust with cancer.*

What You Can Expect From Your Health Care Team

You can expect your health care team to:

- Provide information about breast cancer and treatment options,
- Answer your questions in a respectful and understandable way—even when you need to repeat the question several times, in different ways,
- Provide information about other services and resources for people with cancer in your community,
- Explain how to contact them between visits, and
- Explain what kinds of symptoms you should report immediately, e.g., sudden bleeding, fever, etc.

What You Can Do to Help Your Health Care Team

Answer questions honestly and completely and try to be concise. This won't be easy if you feel somewhat embarrassed, but your caregivers are there to help you, not judge you.

If You Have a Problem Talking with Your Doctor

If you have a problem talking with your doctor, there are often ways to improve the situation. Try working out your concerns before deciding that the situation is hopeless. First of all, state your concern as honestly and openly as possible. Here are some opening statements you may want to consider:

- "I'm concerned that we aren't communicating well, and here's why..."
- "I need to be able to talk with you about _____, and I feel like I can't. Can we discuss this?"
- "I realize that you're very busy, but I need very much to discuss _____ at more length. Can we schedule a time to do that?"

♦ "I'm having trouble understanding _____. Can you help me?"

If you need more details after your doctor answers a question, say so. Sometimes it's even helpful to ask the question again in a different way. Unless you tell your doctor that you don't understand something, s/he will usually assume that you do. There's nothing wrong with not understanding the first explanation; just ask for another.

If you want to learn more about your cancer treatment, ask your doctor to suggest some reading materials. If you feel comfortable doing so, learning more about your treatment can also help you become more actively involved in it.

If you are unable to work out the problem during your regular visits with your doctor, ask for a special visit to discuss it. If the issue directly concerns your cancer treatment, go to the meeting with as much knowledge as possible. In the U.S. you can call the American Cancer Society at 1-800-ACS-2345 for more information about cancer. Always tell your doctor where you get your information and then ask for his or her opinion.

Even if you feel frustrated or angry, try to avoid being hostile or accusatory toward your doctor. Much of the time, people will become defensive and withdraw if they feel attacked—a response that will be unhelpful in the long run. State your concerns and questions clearly and honestly, without making accusations.

What should you do if you feel you have done your part but the situation has not improved? You might consider talking with a third party about the problem. The head nurse or your family doctor might be willing to discuss the matter with the doctor. Sometimes this is less stressful than facing the doctor directly, and their help could improve the situation. If not, it may be time to find a new doctor. Don't stay with a doctor only to protect his or her feelings. Just because you were referred to the doctor does not mean you can't decide to change on your own. It's your body and you have the right to find the best doctor for you.

You can also be a partner in the decision making about your treatments. Although the information about cancer can seem overwhelming when you feel time pressing you, a skilled doctor or nurse can simplify the facts so that two or three options can be presented at any time during your treatments. No matter how complex your problems might seem, your health care team can help you through the process.

Lastly, you need to be an active participant in healing—no one else has as much invested in your body as you do! You can help manage the side effects of treatments by paying attention to your sleep, diet, and exercise regime. You can keep a journal of the questions, changes, or symptoms that you notice between visits, keep your appointments, give your team occasional feedback about how you're doing, and use the services and supports that are available at the clinic and in your community.

> *Except on bad chemo days, everyone has to eat. One friend made batches of old-fashioned chicken soup with vegetables in a thick broth. That soup turned out to be all I ate for several days after each treatment.*

COUNSELORS

Doctors and surgeons are trained to deal with tumors, but you are also learning to live with the confusion and pain that follows a diagnosis of cancer. To help you cope with the emotional and spiritual side of cancer, you might want to talk to a nurse, social worker, psychologist, or counselor experienced in the particular problems and challenges cancer brings to our lives. Some cities now even have therapists who specialize in counseling cancer patients and families. The people who you love, particularly your partner, your children, other family members, and friends, also need emotional support to help you and to cope with their own fear.

> I still feel the need to talk to survivors, but never make the contact because, in our city, I would have to initiate such a support group, and I don't have a lot of energy emotionally. If there were such a group, I would join. At times I want to forget about the cancer and pretend it never happened, but it haunts me day and night. I want to deal with the anger and fear in a safe place.

CANCER SURVIVOR GROUPS

> I wholeheartedly believe in self-help groups and feel that our local cancer group is invaluable.

Talking to a woman who, like you, has learned to live with cancer might be helpful and comforting. If you do not already know such a woman, check the Resources section in the back of this book for support groups in your area. Some women have found it helpful to get in touch with such a group or individual before they have any surgery or treatment. The women involved with these groups have had breast cancer and have found their strength again. They will be able to share their experience with you, and many are gentle, informed listeners.

> The bottom line is that once a month I get together with a roomfull of women, all of whom have had breast cancer. And just the air in the room is a relief to breathe.

The most important feature of self-help groups is that the person giving help and the person receiving help are equals—and everyone in the group can do both. Finding that others have the same or similar problems helps group members to feel they are no longer alone. Here are some of the benefits that people in breast cancer groups have talked about:

- Learning more about breast cancer and treatment options
- Learning about available resources such as books, CDs, DVDs, other kinds of groups, clothing, exercise classes, financial help
- Being better able to cope with treatments and side effects: knowing what to expect
- Feeling less fearful
- Being more comfortable talking about having cancer
- Being more able to talk to family, children, and friends
- Feeling stronger
- Feeling better able to make choices
- Being less lonely
- Being more active
- Being more hopeful

Challenges in Breast Cancer Groups

In addition to the benefits of meeting other women in a breast cancer group, there will be challenges as well. Meeting women whose disease is progressing and who might be dying can be heartbreaking. The effects of losses and deaths on other group members can be devastating, especially when members have also become friends. This presents a dilemma for group members. On the one hand is the desire to maintain a hopeful attitude and not overwhelm new members with stories of loss and grief; and on the other is the wish to extend support to members who are seriously ill and to grieve for the friends who die. Groups that have skilled leadership often negotiate these challenges in ways that are helpful, compassionate, and full of grace—and even humor. Without skilled leadership, people might not be able to meet the needs of either the seriously ill members or the newly diagnosed.

By now, you might be thinking that joining a group isn't for you—at least not yet. Maybe you are thinking it could be too painful or that it might remind you too much of your own fears. Perhaps, like most cancer survivors, you would prefer to focus on maintaining a positive attitude and avoid people who are seriously ill, maybe even dying. Again, only you can determine what is right for you and when the time is right (if ever) for you to attend a support group.

> *I am extremely happy and satisfied with my treatment at the cancer center. The one thing missing, however, was any information about support groups. Even now, after four years, I still feel the need to talk to someone other than my family and friends about my cancer.*

OTHER SOURCES OF SUPPORT

> *A loyal friend, with a busy career, dropped off a fresh organic papaya once a week. Another friend, who knew I felt guilty about not eating more veggies, regularly brought me trays of cut vegetables with hummus. It helped when someone didn't ask, "What can I do to help?" but said, "I'll bring dinner this week. Do you want meat loaf or vegetarian lasagne?" That was a question I could answer.*

Nurses, social workers, psychologists, and other types of health care providers can often be helpful to people who are fighting cancer. They might be able to answer your questions about treatment and how you can expect to feel; they can also help you work through the emotional and spiritual issues that may arise from facing cancer. You may be able to find this kind of help by talking with friends or family, asking at your cancer treatment center, or contacting your local breast cancer support group.

> One young woman, the mother of a new baby, phoned to say, "My husband will come over Sunday afternoon with some food. He'll bring the baby so you can meet her, but he won't stay." The baby was adorable and I was left with a basket of black bean soup, chicken curry, couscous, and cranberry loaf. That busy new mum could have guessed I'd turn her down if she'd asked, "What can I do?" She just did something.

A nurse, counselor, social worker, or friend might be able to help you as you work through some of these questions either before or after your surgery:

- What can I do to rebuild my health?
- How will I look after surgery? Will I need a breast prosthesis? How can I decide if I want breast reconstruction?
- Can you show me a picture of what it would look like afterward? (Some women show each other their mastectomy or lumpectomy scars in support groups.)
- How might this affect me sexually?
- What might people say and how will I answer? How might I deal with their concern or their pity?
- How can I deal with the pain?
- What have I learned from the experts I've seen and what is going to work for me, for my life, and for my survival?
- I feel badly about not taking care of my partner, my family, my friends, my job. What can I do?

Friends, family, members of your cultural community, and, possibly, clergy can also help with their love and support. Take what you learn from these people and use it to take charge of your survival!

I was fortunate to have good friends rally round me, not just in the beginning but also throughout. To the ones who left, I can honestly say a gentle goodbye.

FOR FAMILY AND FRIENDS
A List of Some Basic Do's and Don'ts

Do:

- Take your cues from the person with cancer. Some people are very private while others will talk more about their illness. Respect the person's need to share or their need to remain quiet.
- Let them know you care.
- Respect decisions about how the cancer will be treated, even if you disagree.
- Include the person in usual work projects or social events. Let them be the one to tell you if the commitment is too much to manage.
- Listen without always feeling that you have to respond. Sometimes a caring listener is what the person needs the most.
- Expect the person with cancer to have good days and bad days, emotionally and physically.
- Keep your relationship as normal and balanced as possible. While greater patience and compassion are called for during times like these, your colleague should continue to respect your feelings, as you respect his or her feelings.
- Offer to help in concrete, specific ways (see ideas below).

Don't:

- Offer unsolicited advice or be judgmental.
- Feel you must put up with serious displays of temper or mood swings. You shouldn't accept disruptive behavior just because someone is ill.
- Take things too personally. It's normal for the person with cancer to be quieter than usual, to need time alone, and to be angry at times.
- Be afraid to talk about the illness.
- Always feel you have to talk about cancer. The person with cancer may enjoy conversations that don't involve the illness.
- Be afraid to hug or touch your friend if that was a part of your friendship before the illness.
- Be patronizing. (Try not to use a "How sick are you today?" tone when asking how the person is doing.)
- Tell the person with cancer, "I can imagine how you must feel."

WHAT SHOULD I SAY TO THE PERSON WHO HAS CANCER?

It is normal to feel that you don't know what to say to someone who has cancer. You might only know the person casually, or you might have a closer relationship. The most important thing you can do is to acknowledge the situation in some way—whatever is most comfortable for you. You can show interest and concern, you can express encouragement, or you can offer support. Sometimes the simplest expressions of concern are the most meaningful.

Respond from your heart!

Here are some ideas:

- "I'm not sure what to say, but I want you to know I care."
- "I'm sorry to hear that you are going through this."
- "How are you doing?"
- "If you would like to talk about it, I am here."
- "Please let me know if I can help."
- "I'll keep you in my thoughts."

While it is good to be encouraging, it is also important not to show false optimism or to tell the person with cancer to always have a positive attitude. Doing these things may be seen as discounting their fears, concerns, or sad feelings. It is also tempting to say that you know how the person feels. While you may know this is a trying time, no one can know exactly how the person with cancer feels.

Humor can be an important way of coping. It is also another source of support and encouragement. Let the person with cancer take the lead; it is healthy if they find something funny about a side effect, like hair loss or increased appetite, and you can certainly join them in a good laugh. This can be a great way to relieve stress and to take a break from the more serious nature of the situation.

When the person with cancer looks good, let them know! Avoid making comments when their appearance isn't as good, such as "You're looking pale," or "You've lost weight." Cancer and its treatments can be very unpredictable. Be prepared for good days and bad days.

It's usually best not to tell the person with cancer stories about family members or friends who have had cancer. Everyone is different, and these stories may not be helpful. Instead, it is better simply to tell them you know something about cancer because you've been through it with someone else.

MAINTAINING HOPE

Maintaining hope in the face of serious illness helps you to cope with the treatments and side effects. Nurturing your spirit by focusing on the present day rather than on the uncertain future or past worries can be a challenge, but it will make a big difference in your ability to deal with each day. Hope can also be affected by those around you and how they are reacting—especially helpful are people who are good listeners and can offer practical help with housework, transportation, child care and good humor! All of these things can help you avoid or reduce anxiety, depression, and fear.

SUMMARY

You are the most important person on your cancer care team. You are the one who must design your own treatment plan based on what you learn about your disease and from talking to others. Surround yourself with whoever you need to support yourself through this time, including other women who have been through what you are going through.

I'm learning to live with fear—and reach for support. I watch a lot more sunsets and do a lot less housework.

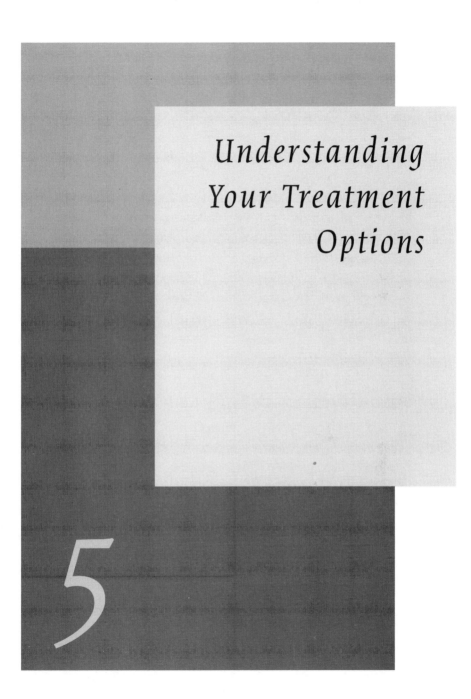

Understanding
Your Treatment
Options

5

This chapter will discuss the next steps in helping you to understand and choose your treatment options.

> For family and friends, it's important to remember what the patient is going through. During treatments your friends might not be themselves. There are massive biochemical changes going on inside them. At times I was weepy, cranky, depressed and judgmental. Be prepared for these changes, bear with your friends and assure them that their wonderful personalities will return soon. Having treatments for cancer was one of the hardest things I've ever had to do; having friends who knew what they could do to help me was one the greatest blessings of my life.
>
> —BERYL YOUNG

How Do I Choose?

There are many different approaches to the treatment of breast cancer, including surgery, with or without radiation, often in combination with chemotherapy and other drug treatments. This chapter will explain what some of the many treatments are, when they are appropriate, and how to weigh the risks and benefits of each choice. These decisions will be based upon the information you already have about your type of cancer, the pathology report, your age, other health factors, and your preferences.

One important source of information is the "Canadian Clinical Practice Guidelines for the Care and Treatment of Breast Cancer" published by the *Canadian Medical Association Journal* (CMAJ). To receive a copy, contact the Cancer Information Service at 1-888-939-3333 or on the Web at www.breastcancerguide.ca. In the U.S., visit the National Cancer Institute Web site at www.nci.nih.gov. Treatment guidelines and patient decision tools can also be found at the National Comprehensive Cancer Network Web site: www.nccn.org.

The information contained in this chapter is targeted to women who have already had a biopsy, know they have breast cancer, and are now considering what to do next. Once you have been diagnosed, there are a number of decisions concerning which treatment or combination of treatments will offer you the best possibility of a long and healthy survival. Remember, there is no single right treatment for everyone. Your breast cancer treatment choices will depend on many factors.

> *Canada and the United States offer some of the best cancer treatment in the world. But in an increasingly complex medical system, women must be aggressive, skeptical, sharp, and savvy consumers to make sure they get the best treatment for them. At the very moment when they see their lives falling apart, when mortality looms large, they must turn themselves into shrewd shoppers.*

Treatment Options

Treatments for breast cancer are generally divided into two categories: local treatment of the breast or lymph gland regions, such as radiation and surgery, and systemic treatment for the rest of the body, such as chemotherapy and/or endocrine or hormone therapy. In addition, there are some unconventional therapies that some people choose to complement traditional cancer therapy.

Many qualitative and quantitative factors will play into the decision/s you and your doctors make regarding treatment. Some women will put more emphasis on quality-of-life issues, others might opt for improved survival rates at any cost.

FERTILITY ISSUES

Premenopausal women who want to have a child after breast cancer treatment should discuss this with their oncologist *before* starting treatment. Chemotherapy affects the entire body, and damage to the reproductive system, and subsequent infertility, is a potential side effect. Ask your oncologist about the likelihood of infertility associated with your treatment options. As mentioned in chapter four, the Clinical Practice Guideline "ASCO Recommendations on Fertility Preservation in People Treated for Cancer" is now available online at www.asco.org.

LOCAL TREATMENTS: SURGERY

Almost all women with breast cancer will have some type of surgery. The type of surgery will depend on a number of things that you should discuss with your surgeon. You will probably have your initial surgery at a local hospital, depending on where your surgeon works. Usually the most convenient choice is the center closest to home.

Choosing a surgeon

You want to have the best outcome from your breast surgery and finding a surgeon will likely start with your family doctor. The ideal surgeon will be experienced and skilled at breast surgery, and someone with whom you feel confident. Your oncologist—if you have seen an oncologist before your surgery—sees a lot of patients after biopsy and other breast surgeries, and can advise you about surgeons who have good surgical technique and whose patients come to the oncologist with "clean margins." (Clean margins indicate that the entire area of breast cancer tissue was cleanly removed and the remaining tissue is free of cancer.)

Surgeons do not always have a warm and friendly bedside manner. While they might not provide you with emotional comfort, they should answer your questions and provide understandable information.

There are several types of surgery for breast cancer. Your operation will depend on the type of cancer you have, the location and size of the tumor, your personal preferences, other medical conditions you might have, and the advice of your surgeon. Some women will have more than one tumor and it might be necessary to remove all of the breast in order to ensure the best outcome. You should take time to understand the options and, if you feel you need to, get a second opinion. Don't let fear and anxiety push you into making a decision until you are ready—breast cancer surgery is not usually a medical emergency and you'll feel better in the long term if you use this time to carefully consider options.

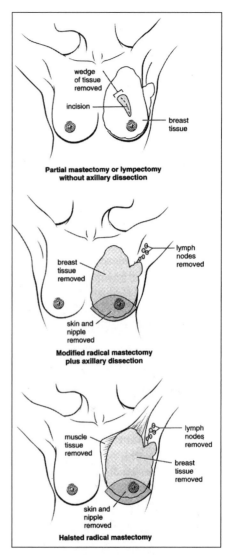

FIGURE 5.1 *Three types of surgery*

Whenever possible, the choice about what surgery is best for you should be based upon your personal preference. Women who are given the choice about what kind of surgery to have adjust better and suffer less anxiety in the long term than women who are told they must have a particular kind of surgery.

Most breast surgeries are done in a hospital under a general anesthetic and require a stay in hospital of one to two days to monitor your recovery.

Simple (Total) Mastectomy

Simple mastectomy surgery will include the removal of all the breast tissue and nipple that normally fits into your bra. The surgeon does not remove any of the underlying chest muscles—the pectoralis major or the pectoralis minor. The lymphatic tissue in your armpit and shoulder area is also not removed.

Modified Radical Mastectomy

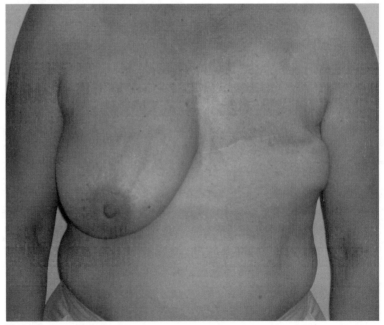

Photo: Dr. M. Levine

UNDERSTANDING YOUR TREATMENT OPTIONS

The Halstead radical mastectomy is the removal of the entire breast, nipple, chest wall muscle beneath the breast, and some of the underarm or axillary lymph nodes. Modified radical mastectomy removes the breast, nipple, and lymph nodes and leaves the chest muscle intact. Modified radical mastectomy has proven as effective as the more radical surgery. It is called "modified" because it removes less of the muscle and lymph tissue.

Mastectomy is a good choice for women who:

- Are not able to have radiation treatment after lumpectomy
- Have large tumors or multiple sites of tumor in a small breast
- Have a high risk of recurrence in the same breast
- Have a personal preference for mastectomy

Radical mastectomies are rarely done today, but if the tumor is large and has invaded the tissue in the chest wall, it might be recommended.

> I went into the hospital in 1946 for what the doctors thought was a small benign lump, but which turned out to be a malignant tumor. I had a child a year and a half later and have been married to a wonderful man for fifty years. I think that things have come a long way since. I do not regret that a complete radical was done, as I have never worried about it since. They also did not give you many choices in the Good Old Days.

Partial Mastectomy/Lumpectomy/Segmental Mastectomy/Wide-Excision

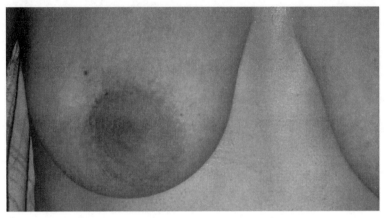

Photo: Dr. M. Levine

The alternative to mastectomy is a surgery that removes only the cancerous section and a margin of the surrounding normal breast tissue. Standard treatment following a partial mastectomy or lumpectomy is radiation treatment. Partial mastectomy, lumpectomy, breast-conserving surgery, wide excision, segmental mastectomy, and quadrantectomy are all names you might hear used for this operation. The part removed can be anywhere from 1 percent to 25 percent of the breast tissue. The intent is to remove the cancerous tissue, paying careful attention to the "margins"—the edges of the tumor between the cancerous tumor and the healthy tissue, allowing enough tissue for the breast to look normal. In almost all cases, four to six weeks of radiation therapy will follow surgery.

There are some women who should not have a lumpectomy:

- Women who have had previous radiation treatment to the chest or breast
- Women with two or more areas of cancer in the same breast

UNDERSTANDING YOUR TREATMENT OPTIONS

- Women with connective tissue disorders that make them sensitive to radiation and may prevent them from healing
- Pregnant women

For women who have a lumpectomy, it is important to know if the margins of the lumpectomy specimen are "clear" or free of cancer. Sometimes the surgeon won't know this until a pathologist has examined the specimen. The surgeon generally takes a wide margin around the tumor; nonetheless, the surgeon cannot see what is going on at the cellular level.

Women should ask the surgeon if the tumor margins were clear. Sometimes a patient will arrive to see her oncologist, assuming that the tumor was clear, only to find out that more surgery or an extra "boost" of radiation to the tumor bed might be needed.

If you have a partial mastectomy or lumpectomy, you will likely have radiation afterwards to reduce the risk of recurrence. Radiation treatment may be difficult for some women because of other medical problems such as lung disease or severe heart disease, age, difficulty traveling long distances to the clinic for daily radiation for four to six weeks. You might consider having a modified radical mastectomy if these are problems for you.

Tomorrow will be "look at my bare chest" day. I have been protected by bandages for a week. Now I must face the fact. I have but one breast. And a scar. Some champagne perhaps? To celebrate the new image.

—BARB SULLIVAN,
My Broken Breast Book

Axillary Lymph Node Dissection or Sentinel Node Biopsy

The surgeon might also remove fat and lymph nodes from the armpit area to find out if there are any cancer cells spreading beyond the breast tissue. The lymph nodes are part of the system that carries fluid, called "lymph," around the body. When breast cancer spreads, it often collects in the lymph nodes in the armpit area. By surgically removing the nodes and examining them microscopically, the pathologist can determine if the nodes are "positive" (containing cancer cells) or "negative" (no cancer cells). There are three levels of lymph nodes in the armpit area. The surgeon usually removes the lowest and midaxillary-level nodes.

Rather than removing all or most of the underarm lymph nodes, a "sentinel node" biopsy might be considered. During a sentinel node biopsy, radioactive material or a dye (or both) is injected into the breast tissue surrounding the tumor. As the lymph carries the dye through the lymphatic pathways, the surgeon uses a device that identifies whether the first lymph node—the sentinel node—is free of cancer. If it is, then no other lymph nodes need to be removed and the surgery has minimal side effects. The sentinel lymph node is thought to accurately reflect the state of all of the nodes in the armpit. There is always a small chance that even though no cancer cells are found in the sentinel node, some cancer cells may be hidden in other nodes; this can affect the success of treatments. If the sentinel lymph node is found to contain cancer cells, the surgeon will go on to perform an axillary node dissection.

Side effects of these operations include temporary swelling and tenderness and hardness due to scar tissue that forms in the surgical site.

Choosing between lumpectomy and mastectomy: The advantage of lumpectomy is that it saves the appearance of the breast. A disadvantage is the need for several weeks of radiation therapy after surgery. However, a small percentage of women who have a mastectomy still need radiation therapy to the breast area.

In determining the preference for lumpectomy or mastectomy, be sure to obtain all the facts. Though you might have an initial gut feeling for mastectomy to "take it all out as quickly as possible," the fact is that doing so does not provide any better chance of long-term survival or a better outcome from treatment in most cases. Large research studies with thousands of women participating and more than twenty years of accumulated information show that when lumpectomy can be performed, mastectomy does not provide any better chance of survival from breast cancer than lumpectomy; because of these facts, most women do not have the breast removed. Also, women who undergo lumpectomy and radiation still have a small chance of the cancer returning in the breast. If this happens, it can be very upsetting, but there are many effective treatments for this.

Although most women and their doctors prefer lumpectomy and radiation therapy, your choice will depend on a number of factors, such as:

+ How you feel about losing your breast
+ How far you have to travel for radiation therapy
+ Whether you are willing to have more surgery to reconstruct your breast after having a mastectomy
+ Your preference for mastectomy as a way to get rid of all your cancer as quickly as possible

What Will Surgery Be Like?

Depending on the type of surgery you have and how soon you recover, your hospital stay could last only one or two days. The length of your stay might also depend on the region of the country you live in. You are usually asked to check into the hospital early, on the same day as your surgery. The doctor who administers the anesthesia (anesthesiologist) will likely visit you briefly and should answer any questions you may ask. Let the anesthesiologist know if you have had problems, such as nausea, vomiting, severe or unusual pain, or other side effects with previous surgery and recovery; or if a close blood relative has had any difficulties with an anesthetic. You will not be allowed to eat or drink from the evening before the surgery until after you have been brought back from the recovery room.

Depending on the type of surgery, the operation will likely take from two to four hours. Following surgery, your breast will be bandaged and one or two tubes will be in place to drain fluid from the wound. Your throat might be sore from the airway tube that was in place during surgery. You might feel sick to your stomach and tired; and there might be numbness, tingling, or pain in your chest, shoulder, or arm. Some women feel pain in the breast they have lost. If you are in pain, you can ask for medication. It is important for you to rest after the surgery and regain your strength.

After the surgery, you will probably want to have someone nearby who cares about you and who can speak to the surgeon. Make sure that person's name and phone number is clearly written in your chart. The surgeon might want to talk to him or her (when you are in the recovery room) to describe what was found during the operation.

Among the possible short-term side effects of both mastectomy and lumpectomy are:

+ Wound infection
+ Hematoma or blood that accumulates in the wound
+ Seroma or accumulation of clear fluid in the wound, which can be drained

Long-term effects can include:

- Pain or "postmastectomy syndrome" that is caused by nerve damage
- Lymphedema or swelling caused by removal of the lymph glands, which can happen even years after surgery

Medication can help manage the pain rapidly and completely. Compression and massage can help manage chronic pain from lymphedema. And there are alternative therapies, such as meditation, biofeedback, yoga, prayer, visualization, tai chi, therapeutic touch, and herbal remedies. Although there is not sufficient scientific evidence about these therapies, many patients report significant benefits.

Pain can also be caused by the emotional distress of a cancer diagnosis and can be made worse because of fear, anxiety, or depression. Talking to friends, family, support group members, or professional counselors can help you to manage this difficult time.

Shortly after surgery, when you have had some time to rest, your surgeon will probably meet with you to discuss the surgery. Your surgeon might comment on the amount of tissue removed and the number of lymph nodes sent to the lab for biopsy. The results of the lymph node biopsy will help determine the stage of your disease.

You will also have one or two tubes in the area around the surgical wound. The drains stay in place for several days, to prevent fluids from accumulating, and are removed within a few days of the surgery.

If, for any reason, you must remain in hospital for several days, your family and friends might be anxious to visit. You might find visitors to be a help—or maybe not. Some visitors might need more help than you do—don't let them use up your energy. Consider telling *only* close friends and family that you are going into the hospital; this will provide the quiet time you need to heal and adjust.

Before Leaving the Hospital

This is often a very difficult time as you wait for the pathology reports. The amount of time it will take for the pathology results to come back can vary greatly from one hospital to another and one region to the next. Some women find this to be a particularly difficult time, as they wonder and worry about the future, imagining all kinds of things happening to them. You might find it helpful to talk to your nurses and caregivers about your feelings. You might want to talk with someone from your local breast cancer support group, if there is one in your area. They can arrange a hospital or home visit, a group meeting, or provide support by telephone.

> *The time it took for the diagnosis to be available after the lumpectomy was especially long—almost one week. It was the longest week in my life. Maybe my case was exceptional, but anything done to speed up the time would have been appreciated.*

Before you leave the hospital, you should be shown how to care for your surgical wound. Ask when it is all right to shave or use deodorant (most deodorants contain aluminum, which might interfere with radiation treatments). Ask when the stitches will be removed.

Before you go home, discuss with your doctor how you will take care of the surgical wound and arm. Written instructions about care after surgery are usually given to you and your caregivers. These instructions should include:

- how to care for the surgical wound and dressing
- how to monitor drainage and take care of the drains
- how to recognize signs of infection
- when to call the doctor or nurse and the phone numbers to contact them

- when to begin using the arm and how to do arm exercises to prevent stiffness
- when to resume wearing a bra
- when to begin using a prosthesis and what type to use (after mastectomy)
- what to eat and not to eat
- use of medications, including pain medicines
- any restrictions of activity
- what to expect regarding sensations or numbness in the breast and surgical arm
- what to expect regarding feelings about body image
- information about a follow-up appointment

Arriving Home

You could arrive home as early as a day or two after surgery, even after a bilateral mastectomy. When you arrive home, have someone available to help out, as you might have trouble lifting your arm(s) for a couple days, and feel weak from the anesthetic. Many hospitals will arrange for a nurse to visit to help you change your drains. Your stitches are usually removed a week after surgery by either your family doctor or your surgeon. Many surgeons use dissolving stitches, which don't need to be removed.

Two to four weeks might pass before you feel ready to drive or go back to work. Some women have found that shoulder-strap car seat belts are irritating if they rub against the scar. You could try putting a soft cloth between the belt and you.

Oddly enough, the week after my surgery was one of the most social weeks of my life, with people dropping in with flowers, food, and offers of child care. I was really moved by their generosity and it helped me to

let go a little of my tendency to want to control and just accept the care I
needed during one of the hardest weeks of my life.

For a few weeks or more, as the scar heals, you might want to wear soft, loose-fitting clothing. If your surgery was a mastectomy, when the scar has healed you can choose to wear a soft breast, called a "prosthesis," in your bra. Temporary prostheses are often available free of charge from the American or Canadian Cancer societies or from your local support group. If you are not having further treatment (radiation or chemotherapy), you might be able to have breast reconstruction surgery at the same time as your mastectomy or soon after, if you wish. It is wise to discuss this option with your surgeon during your visits before surgery.

Like many women, you might feel comfortable with your changed body just as it is and not choose breast reconstruction. Some women simply don't want to go through any more surgery. There are a number of options you might want to consider. You might need to take some time (and this may be months or years) to become fully comfortable in choosing the right option.

Most patients see their doctor within seven to fourteen days following the surgery. Your doctor should explain the results of your pathology report and talk to you about the need for further treatment. If you will need more treatment, you will be referred to a medical oncologist and/or radiation oncologist.

Keeping Active

Whether you had a mastectomy or lumpectomy, if lymph nodes were removed, your arm might be weak. If physiotherapy is not routinely offered in your hospital, you can request to meet with someone from the rehabilitation or physiotherapy department who is knowledgeable about breast cancer and who will show you exercises that will help regain the strength in your arm and maintain mobility. These exercises are an important part of your recovery and will prevent muscles in the arm and shoulder from becoming "frozen" or stiff. Whether you get help with exercising in the hospital or plan your own exercises, keep active in order to prevent long-term problems with circulation and movement.

Lymphedema

Some women develop a condition called "lymphedema," which is a swelling in the arm or hand because the lymph nodes are not properly draining the lymph fluid. Although it is becoming less common as surgical

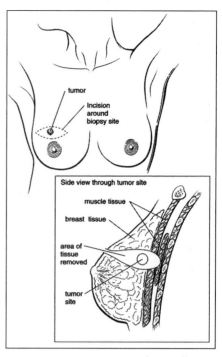

FIGURE 5.2 *Lumpectomy without axillary dissection (no lymph nodes removed)*

techniques become more sophisticated, lymphedema can happen anytime after the surgery (even years later) and it may be temporary or permanent.

> My only regret is lymphedema in my arm. I wish I could get relief from this. It is very annoying during short-sleeve season. Otherwise, I am happy to have had the surgery and I've been healthy ever since. This is all I have to bear.

Some women have also found massage therapy to be helpful for arm problems after surgery. Therapeutic massage by a registered massage therapist (RMT) can help to increase blood flow and lymph flow at

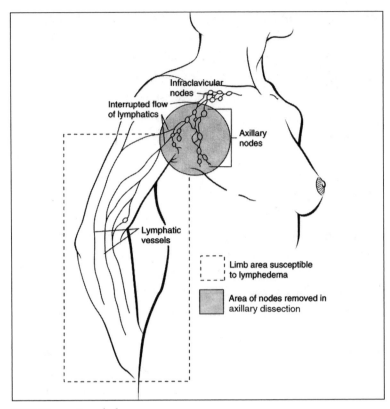

FIGURE 5.3 *Lymphedema*

a time when it will be difficult for you to enjoy these benefits
from exercise.

Many women experience numbness and a change in feeling
around their scar, which sometimes travels through the arm. This is
caused by the nerves that have been cut during surgery and which are
now healing. The numbness might diminish in a year or so, but in
some women it can last longer. You might find it helpful to use a small
soft pillow to support the arm when you are sitting or lying down. The
changed feeling around the surgery site might not always be unpleasant. Some women have reported the feeling as pleasant, even sensual.

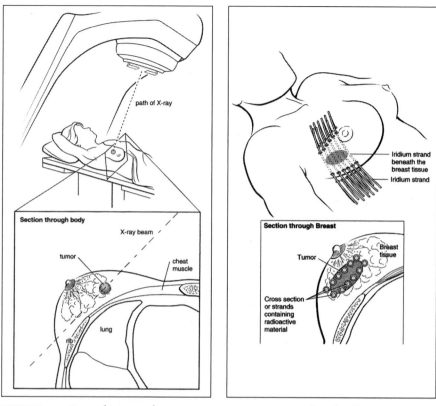

FIGURE 5.4 *How radiation works*

FIGURE 5.5 *Implanted radioisotopes*

LOCAL TREATMENTS: RADIATION THERAPY

A partial mastectomy or a lumpectomy is usually followed by radiation treatment to the breast. Radiation treatment helps prevent a recurrence of cancer in the breast. Although many specialists consider this treatment standard and necessary after surgery, it is important to remember that you have a choice in this.

Radiation therapy following breast-conserving surgery is standard treatment, but occasionally it can be omitted. This should be discussed with your radiation oncologist. Women who might consider lumpectomy without radiation therapy have all of the following:

- age seventy years or older
- a tumor 2 cm or less that has been completely removed
- a tumor that contains hormone receptors
- no lymph node involvement

The chance of recurrence is greater in younger women (younger than age forty-six) than older women (older than age seventy), so this factor should be considered, as well.

Radiation therapy takes place five days a week for three to six weeks. Radiation treatment uses high-energy X-rays to kill cancer cells and shrink tumors by heating the cells to a high temperature. Radiation can also cause "sunburn" and red, sore skin. Sometimes an extra amount of radiation treatment is administered to the site of the original tumor. This is called a "boost."

Before your treatments start, the radiation team carefully takes measurements to determine the correct angles for aiming the radiation beams and the proper dose of radiation. They will make some ink marks or small tattoos on your skin that they will use later as a guide to focus the radiation on the right area. Deodorants and antiperspirants can interfere with external beam radiation therapy of the underarm area, so you should avoid using them until treatments are complete.

External radiation is done by machines that direct the X-rays to precise areas of the body, such as a part of the breast. This is the type of radiation that most women receive. Radiation treatments affect only the area to which the X-rays are directed.

Brachytherapy, also known as internal radiation, is another way to deliver radiation therapy. A small number of women receive this type of radiation. Instead of aiming radiation beams from outside the body, radioactive seeds or pellets are placed directly into the breast tissue next to the cancer. Sometimes, this method is used in addition to external breast radiation, but more often is used to give an extra "boost" of radiation to the tumor site. This method is being studied in clinical trials. So far, the results have been promising, but more experience is needed with this technique before it can be recommended as standard treatment.

Recently, new techniques, called accelerated partial breast irradiation, of delivering high doses of radiation to the tumor site have been used. Other types of local accelerated breast irradiation treatment are being studied in clinical trials. Although they appear promising, the long-term benefits and side effects remain to be determined. Methods of delivering this type of treatment include:

+ Mammosite radiation therapy system
+ 3D conformal external beam
+ Intra-operative

Because radiation therapy treatments require the use of sophisticated and expensive machinery, they are usually only available in specialized cancer centers and certain hospitals. Therefore, you might have to travel on a daily basis or stay away from home for a period of three to six weeks to receive your radiation treatments. Many cancer centers make arrangements to assist patients with daily travel (volunteer drivers) or overnight stays (such as lodge accommodations). Ask the staff at the treatment center if you can take advantage of this assistance.

For women who have the following health conditions, radiation therapy is not a good choice:

+ pregnancy
+ previous radiation treatment to the breast or chest area
+ arthritis that prevents you from lying flat for a long period with arms extended

- systemic lupus erythematosus
- scleroderma

SYSTEMIC ADJUVANT TREATMENTS

If, after surgery, your lymph nodes show that the cancer has spread, or there are other worrisome features of the tumor, your doctor should discuss systemic treatments with you. Systemic treatments are used to treat cancer throughout the body, in every cell. Ask questions and consider getting the opinion of a medical oncologist if further treatment is recommended for you. When patients who have no detectable cancer after surgery are given systemic therapy, it is called adjuvant therapy. The goal of adjuvant therapy is to kill hidden cells that might be present but are undetected. Not every patient needs adjuvant therapy, however. Generally speaking, if the tumor is larger than one-half inch or the cancer has spread to lymph nodes or if it is high grade, it is more likely to have spread through the bloodstream elsewhere in the body.

For large tumors, chemotherapy or radiation is sometimes given before surgery to shrink the size (this is called neo-adjuvant treatment). In this case, you might be referred to an oncologist before surgery, or you might ask for a referral before deciding on treatment.

Chemotherapy

Chemotherapy uses drugs, taken by injection or in pill form, to kill cancer cells. The drugs work by preventing the cells from dividing or reproducing, which forces them to die. But the drugs are not very selective. They will kill many other healthy cells that are also dividing, including hair cells and bone marrow cells. This explains why some women lose their hair during chemotherapy treatments. In bone marrow, the drugs lower the body's production of red and white blood cells and platelets. This can affect your energy level, your ability to fight off infection, and the ability of your blood to clot properly. Remember that these effects are only temporary. Your blood cells will begin to function normally once you have stopped having treatments.

Research has shown that chemotherapy drugs are more effective when used in combination rather than singly. The most frequently used combinations are:

- Cyclophosphamide (Cytoxan), methotrexate (Amethopterin, Mexate, Folex), and fluorouracil (Fluorouracil, 5-FU, Adrucil) [CMF]
- Fluorouracil, doxorubicin (Adriamycin), and cyclophosphamide [FAC]
- Doxorubicin (Adriamycin) and cyclophosphamide [AC]
- Doxorubicin (Adriamycin) and cyclophosphamide followed by paclitaxel (Taxol) or docetaxel (T) [ACT]
- Docetaxel, doxorubicin, cyclophosphamide [TAC]
- Doxorubicin (Adriamycin), followed by CMF
- Cyclophosphamide, epirubicin (Ellence), and fluorouracil with or without docetaxel

Doctors give chemotherapy in cycles, with each period of treatment followed by a rest period. The chemotherapy is given on the first day of each cycle, and then the body is given time to recover from the effects of chemotherapy. The chemotherapy drugs are then repeated to start the next cycle. The time between giving the chemotherapy drugs is generally every two weeks, or every three weeks. Some drugs are given more often. When given as adjuvant therapy, these cycles generally last for a total time of three to six months, depending on the drugs used.

Chemotherapy is usually given following the initial treatment of surgery and radiation. Chemotherapy treatments are usually given in specialized cancer treatment centers, but can also be administered through community clinics or hospital outpatient departments. The location will depend on where you live and which oncologist you see. Be sure to advise your dentist, chiropractor, or other health care providers that you are in chemotherapy treatment. You should arrange a dental checkup before starting chemotherapy to avoid any bleeding problems caused by the drugs.

High-Dose Chemotherapy with Autologous Bone Marrow or Peripheral Blood Stem Cell Support

Although it is possible to use very high doses of chemotherapy or radiation to kill cancer cells, such treatments also kill blood-producing stem cells in the bone marrow. Damage to bone marrow stem cells lowers the white blood cell count, which makes the patient very vulnerable to potentially fatal infections and bleeding.

One way to get around this is to remove some of the patient's stem cells from either the peripheral (circulating) blood or bone marrow and then return them into a vein after high-dose chemotherapy. The stem cells are able to find the bone marrow and soon reestablish themselves and restore the body's ability to produce blood cells.

It was thought that this would be a good way to treat women whose breast cancer was diagnosed at an advanced stage, for example, if they had many lymph nodes involved. Several studies evaluating this treatment have showed no benefit. Women who received the high-dose chemotherapy did not live any longer than women who received standard-dose chemotherapy without stem cell support.

High-dose chemotherapy with stem cell support also causes more serious side effects than standard-dose chemotherapy. Research in this area is still being conducted. Recent studies found that in certain women whose cancer had spread to many lymph nodes, high-dose chemotherapy did not lower the death rate. Although newer studies may show a drop in death rate, it will likely be very small. And the toxicity from this treatment is very high. Experts in the field now recommend that women not receive high-dose chemotherapy except as part of a clinical trial.

Monoclonal Antibody Therapy with Trastuzumab (Herceptin®)

Antibodies are proteins produced by immune system cells that attach to certain chemicals that the body recognizes as not being part of its own normal tissues. Antibodies help your body resist infections, and even cancer. Monoclonal antibodies are a special type of antibody that can be mass-produced in laboratories.

Trastuzumab (Herceptin®) is a monoclonal antibody that attaches to a growth-promoting protein known as HER2/neu, which is present in small amounts on the surface of normal breast cells and most breast cancers. About one-quarter of breast cancers have too much of this protein and tend to grow and spread more aggressively. Trastuzumab can prevent the HER2/neu protein from making breast cancer cells grow and may also stimulate the immune system to more effectively attack the cancer.

Herceptin® can shrink some breast cancer metastases that return after chemotherapy or continue to grow during chemotherapy. In some patients, treatment that combines Herceptin® with chemotherapy might be more effective than chemotherapy alone.

Recently, clinical trials have been completed that found that adding trastuzumab at the end of the chemotherapy regimen lowers the recurrence rate and death rate over chemotherapy alone after surgery in women with HER2/neu positive early breast cancers. Now in both Canada and the United States trastuzumab is routinely given at the end

Adjuvant Breast Cancer Treatment Options for Patients

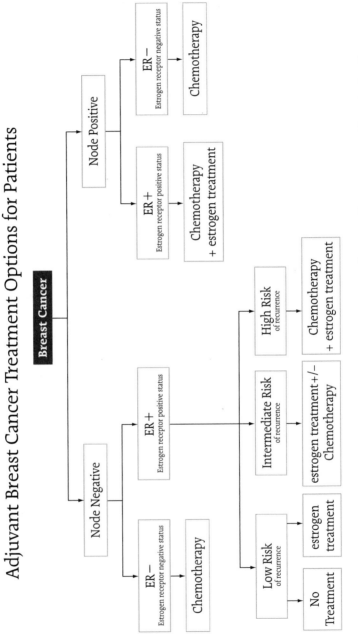

Adapted from: Abraham eds., et al. *Bethesda Handbook of Clinical Oncology*. Lippincott, Williams & Wilkins, 2001, 13; and from the Canadian Guidelines for node negative and node positive breast cancer in the CMAJ.

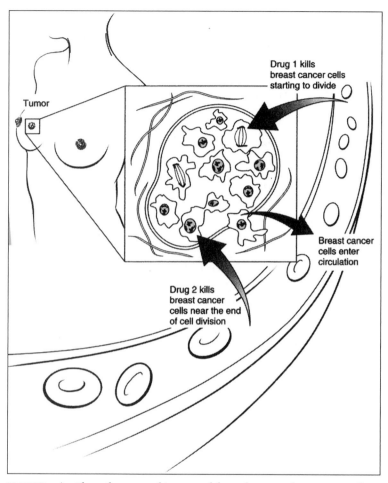

FIGURE 5.6   *Chemotherapy combines several drugs that act on breast cancer cells at different stages of cell division.*

of chemotherapy in women whose tumors overexpress HER2/neu.

Compared with chemotherapy drugs, the side effects of trastuzumba are relatively mild. They can include fever and chills, and headache. These side effects are usually associated with the first dose and do not recur. Some women being treated with trastuzumab, however, have experienced heart damage leading to congestive heart failure. In the research studies using this drug after chemotherapy regimens containing adriamycin or epirubicin the risk of congestive heart failure was between 1 and 3 percent. For some women, this effect on the heart is temporary and improves when the drug is stopped. Major symptoms are shortness of breath and severe fatigue. Women experiencing these symptoms should call their doctor right away.

While you are receiving trastuzumab, your doctor will arrange for you to have a heart scan about every three months to monitor how your heart is functioning. If there is a drop in the functioning of the heart, the medication will be stopped.

Ask your oncologist to explain your particular chemotherapy treatment to you. The side effects will depend on the type of drugs used, the length of treatment, and the amount taken.

Endocrine (Hormone) Therapy

Until menopause, the hormone estrogen is produced mainly by a woman's ovaries. Estrogen promotes the growth of about two-thirds of breast cancers (those containing estrogen or progesterone receptors). Because of this, several approaches to blocking the effect of estrogen or lowering estrogen levels are used to treat breast cancer.

If your breast cancer is identified as hormone-sensitive (that is, estrogen or progesterone positive) you might benefit from endocrine therapy, which starts after chemotherapy and radiation are finished. There are two main endocrine therapy options: Tamoxifen and aromatase inhibitors.

Tamoxifen Medications such as tamoxifen (Nolvadex) block the estrogen receptor that is a docking site on the cancer cell to which estrogen sticks—causing a signal to be transmitted to the nucleus of the cell that causes it to grow. Tamoxifen will bind to the estrogen receptor, thus blocking the estrogen uptake by the cancer cell. Hence, the growth of certain estrogen-sensitive tumors is reduced. The side effects of these drugs might not be as harsh as chemotherapy, but their purpose is the same: to keep cancer cells from growing.

Tamoxifen is often used as an adjuvant therapy option for both pre- and postmenopausal women with hormone receptor positive early-stage breast cancer. It is generally taken for five years and then stopped, as there is no evidence that extending this period has any survival benefit.

The most common side effects of tamoxifen, include hot flashes, endometrial carcinoma irregular periods, and vaginal discharge. In less than 1 percent of cases, it increases the risk of developing blood clots in the legs and lungs.

Aromatase Inhibitors A relatively new class of hormone-modifying drugs, called aromatase inhibitors, has been used for a number of years in women with advanced breast cancer. Recently a number of trials have demonstrated their value in early breast cancer in preventing the recurrence of breast cancer. They include anastrozole (Arimidex), letrozole (Femara), and exemestane (Aromasin). Unlike tamoxifen, which works by blocking the binding of estrogen to the cancer cell, aromatase inhibitors actually cause a marked reduction in the amount of estrogen your body produces. They work by blocking an enzyme, aromatase, responsible for producing small amounts of estrogen in postmenopausal women—who can generate estrogen in fat tissue, the breasts and the adrenal glands. They cannot stop the ovaries of premenopausal women from producing estrogen. For this reason they are effective only in postmenopausal women, especially those with ER-positive cancer. The most significant side effect is the greater risk of osteoporosis (and bone fractures) caused by bone loss associated with lower estrogen levels. Mild side effects include hot flashes (less so than with tamoxifen), joint pain, muscle aches, and fatigue. Aromatase inhibitors have fewer side effects than tamoxifen because they don't cause endometrial cancer and very rarely cause blood clots.

Aromatase inhibitors have been compared with tamoxifen as adjuvant hormone therapy in postmenopausal women with early breast cancer and have shown an advantage. Clinical trials continue to assess a number of strategies that explore how best to use these drugs.

OOPHORECTOMY

Nowadays, a less common treatment for estrogen receptor positive breast cancer patients is the removal of the ovaries, or oophorectomy, which removes the woman's primary source of estrogen. This treatment was common before the development of anti-estrogen drugs like tamoxifen, and is still occasionally recommended for women who are premenopausal. Oopherectomy can be done surgically, or medically with a drug called Zoledex. There is some evidence that premenopausal women with breast cancer, who continue to menstruate after chemotherapy, have a worse prognosis than those whose periods stop. There are ongoing trials examining whether the addition of Zoledex in such women will improve their outcomes.

LOCALLY ADVANCED BREAST CANCER

Patients with locally advanced breast cancer (LABC) have large breast tumors (more than 5 cm wide) and one or more of the following:

+ Tumors that are attached to the chest wall or skin, or skin that is ulcerated or red

- Lymph nodes under the arm that have become attached to structures under the arm
- Lymph nodes above the collarbone (supraclavicular nodes) that contain cancer cells

Inflammatory breast cancer, which makes the breast red and swollen, is a type of LABC. The inflammation occurs because the lymphatic channels in the skin of the breast are blocked by tumor cells, which results in edema (excessive accumulation of fluid) of the breast.

The treatment of LABC is complex and must be tailored to the patient. Patients will often need a combination of therapies (combined modality treatment). This includes chemotherapy, mastectomy, and radiation.

In the management of LABC, it is very important that the surgeon, medical oncologist, and radiation oncologist work together to plan treatment.

Usually, LABC is not operable because the cancer is too big and/or fixed to underlying structures. Chemotherapy that usually includes anthracyclines and taxanes is given in order to shrink the tumor. If the cancer responds well to the chemotherapy—i.e., shrinks to at least half the original size—then treatment will usually continue for four to six months. When and if the tumor shrinks and is freely mobile, then surgery, consisting of a mastectomy and axillary node dissection, is performed. Then the patient is offered local regional radiation therapy, which generally includes the chest wall, the lymph nodes under the arm and above the collarbone. If the tumor is estrogen receptor therapy positive, then endocrine therapy is also used.

UNCONVENTIONAL THERAPIES

More and more people in North America are looking to unconventional therapies not only to prevent illness but also to help them recover from illness. Complementary and alternative therapies are a diverse group of health care practices, systems, and products that are not part of usual medical treatment. They could include products such as vitamins, herbs, or dietary supplements, or procedures such as acupuncture, massage, and a host of other types of treatment. Many are now being studied to find out if they are truly helpful to people with cancer.

You might hear about different treatments from family, friends, and others that could be offered as a way to treat your cancer or to help you feel better. Some of these treatments are harmless in certain situations, while others have been shown to cause harm. Most of them are of unproven benefit.

The American Cancer Society defines complementary medicine or methods as those that are used along with your regular medical care. If these treatments are carefully managed, they may add to your comfort and well-being. Alternative medicines are defined as those that are used instead of your regular medical care. Some of them have been proven not to be useful or even to be harmful, but are still promoted as "cures." If you choose to use these alternatives, they may reduce your chance of fighting your cancer by delaying, replacing, or interfering with regular cancer treatment.

Many of these therapies have not been put through rigorous scientific testing to prove whether or not they are effective. Also, as many cancer patients have learned, medical doctors sometimes view them as quackery. It is important to remember, however, that many of the treatments we have come to view as standard cancer care (such as radiation) were also once viewed as quackery and dismissed by the medical profession. Some medical doctors view any unconventional therapies as useless because their effectiveness has not been scientifically proven.

You can find out more about complementary and alternative therapies on the Web at the National Center for Complementary and Alternative Medicine (NCCAM) at www.nccam.nih.gov. The NCCAM is an advocate for quality science, rigorous and relevant research, and open and objective inquiry into which complementary and alternative medicines (CAM) practices work, which do not, and why. Its overriding mission is to give the public reliable information about the safety and effectiveness of CAM practices.

> Modern medicine has largely focused on the physical side of the problem, aggressively attacking the illness, often ignoring the person who has it. On the other hand, alternative medicine has focused on the person rather than the disease, insisting that it is simply mind over matter: fix it in your mind and the physical problem will take care of itself. This approach is equally wrong. It is the interaction of the mind and body that matters. Coping with illness is both a mental and physical process.
>
> —DR. DAVID SPIEGEL, *Living Beyond Limits: New Hope and Help for Facing Life-Threatening Illness*

There was a time when the foods we ate were not seen to play a role in the development of cancer. We now know from research that certain types of food eaten on a regular basis—like broccoli, cauliflower, and Brussels sprouts—can help prevent the development of certain types of cancer. As well, some unconventional therapies gaining popularity in Western countries today have been used for centuries in other cultures and countries, such as herbal remedies and acupuncture. The health care community's understanding of which unconventional treatments work and which don't is continually evolving.

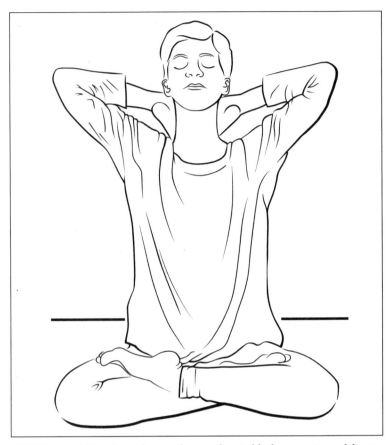

FIGURE 5.7   *Self-healing techniques focus on the mind-body connection and directing the body's own spiritual energy towards healing*

Remember, it is important not to abandon potentially helpful conventional therapies if you also plan to explore unconventional ones.

> *It's heartbreaking when women die of breast cancer because they were too scared to take chemotherapy and radiation. As in my case, these aggressive treatments were highly successful against breast cancer. There is a complementary role, however, for alternative therapies to help us*

UNDERSTANDING YOUR TREATMENT OPTIONS

regain and maintain our well-being—and to help prevent illness in the first place. But it is very confusing for people to distinguish what is useful when conventional practitioners are unwilling to consider anything that doesn't come from pharmaceutical companies. I've found value in many dietary, herbal, and vitamin supports, and in exercise, visualization, and progressive relaxation. More openness about complementary aids might help people to not chase the rainbow of "miracle cures" that do no more than drain financial resources, while also increasing individual responsibility for our health.

Our mental and spiritual states are linked in very important ways to the physical workings of our bodies. There is a belief that the mind can help to heal the body and promote well-being. Techniques that focus on the mind–body connection include meditation, relaxation techniques, laughter therapy, and visualization. These techniques can reduce the pain and uncomfortable side effects of treatment by stimulating the production of endorphins, which are natural painkillers produced in the brain. For some people, prayer has a similar effect.

One of the difficulties that cancer patients face is finding reliable information about unconventional therapies and someone who can help them sort out what they need. Some states and provinces have legislation that governs health care providers who work with certain unconventional therapies; these include naturopaths, acupuncturists, herbalists, massage therapists, chiropractors, and osteopaths. Often you can find out more about unconventional therapies and health care providers who are knowledgeable about them in breast cancer support groups.

If you are interested in pursuing unconventional therapies as part of your cancer treatment, first gather as much information as you can. Then talk about it with your health care team. Patients should not be afraid to discuss alternative therapies with their doctors. There needs to be mutual understanding and respect, and if the patient chooses complementary or alternative therapies, this should not prejudice care. However, if the doctor is not keen, the patient should respect the doctor's expertise.

While it is not yet clear which of the available alternative or complementary therapies can help you physically, we do know that some can certainly help you in a spiritual and emotional sense. Keep in mind that only you can decide what is right for you. Healing is what your body does for itself. Affirming the love and support that is available from family, friends, and ourselves can reduce the helplessness and loneliness brought on by a cancer diagnosis.

Clinical Trials

You may be interested in joining clinical trials of new treatments. Clinical trials are designed by scientists and approved by the U.S. Food and Drug Administration (FDA) and Health Canada to study and compare new treatments with those that have already been proven effective and are available. It was through clinical trials that many of today's standard treatments were proven effective. Computers make the decision about which participants receive the experimental drug and which receive the standard treatment. The experimental drug must be proven to work as effectively, or more effectively, than standard treatments. But it might also have side effects that you and your doctor need to consider along with the potential benefits and risks. The new drug must go through three phases of clinical trials before the FDA or Health Canada considers it for approval.

Phase I   This stage of development focuses on the safety and side effects, the best way to administer the drug, and how much to give. Doctors pay careful attention to side effects and patients are carefully monitored. Drugs in phase I studies have already been proven to be safe in lab studies with animals, but the effects on people are not yet well understood.

Phase II   After the drug's safety has been determined, its effectiveness can be evaluated. Patients are very carefully monitored to determine the drug's effect on the cancer tumor. Baseline studies will be done before you start treatment to measure any changes. Again the side effects are carefully assessed.

Phase III   These are often very large studies with thousands of participants. There will be a "control group" of patients who receive a standard treatment, and another randomly assigned group of patients who receive the "study" or experimental treatment. In this way, researchers can compare the two treatments to find out what differences occur. Again, participants are carefully monitored for side effects and studies can be discontinued if the side effects are severe.

Participating in clinical trials is voluntary, which will be very carefully explained to you and your family. Detailed explanations about the clinical trial will be provided in a written format, along with informed consent documents, which will state that you understand the clinical trial and the potential risks; if you agree to participate in the trial, you must sign the consent forms.

You can leave the study at any time and for any reason. Participating in clinical trials can be an appropriate choice at any stage in your treatment. Although the trial might or might not benefit you directly, clinical trials are the best hope for improving future outcomes for breast cancer patients. You will be carefully monitored and your care and treatment will be as good as (and possibly better than) standard treatments.

SUMMARY

After breast cancer has been confirmed by biopsy, other treatments will follow—likely including some kind of surgery. Radiation may follow the surgery. If there is evidence of disease in the lymph nodes or elsewhere, or if the tumor looks large or aggressive, you will likely have a form of systemic treatment—either chemotherapy or endocrine therapy. Participating in a clinical trial for new treatments is a consideration for all patients.

Anything is one of a million paths. Therefore you must always keep in mind that a path is only a path; if you feel you should not follow it, you must not stay with it under any conditions...Look at every path closely and deliberately. Try it as many times as you think necessary...then ask one question. I will tell you what it is: Does this path have a heart?...If it does, the path is good; if it doesn't, it is of no use.

Both paths lead nowhere; but one has a heart, the other doesn't. One makes for a joyful journey; as long as you follow it, you are one with it. The other will make you curse your life. One makes you strong; the other weakens you...a path without a heart is never enjoyable. You have to work hard even to take it. On the other hand, a path with heart is easy; it does not make you work at liking it...For me there is only the traveling on the paths that have a heart, on any path that may have a heart. There I travel, and the only worthwhile challenge is to traverse its full length. And there I travel—looking, looking, breathlessly.

—CARLOS CASTENADA, *The Teachings of Don Juan:*
A Yaqui Way of Knowledge

Preparing for Treatment and Understanding Side Effects

6

This chapter describes some of the more common physical and emotional side effects of breast cancer treatments and some suggestions about how you can prepare yourself and reduce your discomfort.

> Many people were "just there" for me; making sure I had someone to drive me to each of the chemotherapy treatments, phoning and dropping by with healing lavender oil or ginger tea, staying to empty my dishwasher or fold the laundry that piled up on the end of my bed.
>
> —BERYL YOUNG

Preparing Yourself for Cancer Treatment

Although you will not know exactly what, if any, side effects you might have or how you will feel until after your treatments begin, there are some things you can do to prepare emotionally and practically. This is a time to focus on yourself and on getting well. Here are some ways to get ready:

THINK POSITIVELY

♦ Become well informed about your treatment options—good information can actually help relieve much of your anxiety and fear of the unknown. In the beginning, you might find it helpful to focus on your immediate needs: information about diagnostic tests, treatment options and side effects, appointments, prognosis. Stick with what you need in the moment—don't worry about statistics and data that aren't useful for your decision making: you'll easily become swamped!

- Nurture your sense of hope by concentrating on the present—the past and future are beyond your control, but you do have control over today's decisions and relationships.
- Talk about your feelings with someone you trust and who cares about you—but be cautious with those family members and friends who are very old, very young, or emotionally fragile. They could have difficulty understanding your situation and being supportive, which will put more of a burden on you.
- Develop a good partnership with your health care team—ask questions, record answers, bring a "buddy" along to appointments, expect clear answers. Expect to be treated with respect for yourself as a woman, not a "breast cancer" case—and treat these professionals with the respect they deserve.
- Having cancer and losing a breast can damage a woman's body image, feelings of attractiveness, and chill a couple's intimate, physical relationship. But the good news is that many couples develop a closer bond due to the challenges of breast cancer—let your husband, lover, or partner know how you are feeling and what you need from them.
- Talk to your kids and grandchildren—because they will already sense something is wrong and they might be very frightened. You can help them to understand and experience their sadness and concern in a healthy way; otherwise the secrecy could cause their imaginations to create hurt and the mistaken belief that they are responsible. There are excellent books and other resources to help you talk to your children and grandchildren. (See Resources at the back of this book.)
- Find out if there are support groups or services for newly diagnosed women in your cancer center or community.

- Have a complete dental check-up *before* starting chemotherapy treatment—oral health will be important to your well-being and comfort in eating, should you develop a sore mouth.
- Plan ways to cope with possible side effects from nausea—this can make you feel more in control and help you keep your appetite.
- Many people have few or no side effects that keep them from eating. Even if you have side effects, they may be mild and most go away after cancer treatment ends. In addition, you may be able to control side effects with the new drugs that are available.

A HEALTHY DIET

- A healthy diet is vital for a person's body to function at its best. This is even more important for people with cancer.
- If you maintain a healthy diet, you'll go into treatment with reserves that will help keep up your strength, prevent body tissue from breaking down, rebuild tissue, and maintain your defenses against infection.
- People who eat well are better able to cope with the side effects of treatment. And you may even be able to handle higher doses of certain drugs. In fact, some cancer treatments are more effective in people who are well nourished and are getting enough calories and protein.
- Don't be afraid to try new foods. Some things you might never have liked before could taste good to you during treatment.

Plan Ahead

- Stock the pantry and freezer with your favorite foods so that you won't need to shop as often. Include foods you know you can eat even when you feel sick.

- Cook in advance and freeze foods in meal-sized portions.
- Talk to your friends or family members about helping with shopping and cooking, or ask a friend or family member to take over those jobs for you.
- Let your children, friends, and family know how they can help—you might need to rest and take naps, or need help with driving or cooking, you might feel weepy or cranky—these feelings can frighten family and friends if they aren't prepared. If you and others know to expect these changes, you'll be better able to cope when they flare up.
- Expect some fatigue—and plan to take naps, eat well, and cut back on stressful activities or work.
- Expect some changes with friends—some will be great—others might not. Friends could stop calling for many reasons: they don't know what to say; they are afraid they might hurt your feelings; they are frightened for you and for themselves. Friends can provide various types of support and help at different times along the way—and you'll likely make new friends during your cancer journey.

Stay Fit . . . but Use Caution

Moderate exercise reduces fatigue, promotes a sense of well-being, and can speed recovery from cancer. There might be special precautions you should consider, depending on your treatment or side effects of treatment. For example, if you have severe anemia, you should delay exercise until the anemia has improved. If you are having radiation treatment, you should avoid swimming pools, because chlorine in pool water can be irritating to irradiated skin. If your immune system has been affected by your cancer treatment, you should avoid public gyms (and other public places) until your white blood cell counts return to normal. You should always consult your doctor or nurse before beginning an exercise program.

Should You Use Vitamin and Mineral Supplements?

The best source of vitamins and minerals is found in foods. However, during and just after cancer treatment, you might not eat everything your body needs, so a vitamin and mineral supplement could be required. The best choice is a balanced multivitamin/mineral supplement containing as much as 100 percent of the "Daily Value" of most nutrients (formerly known as the "RDA"). Some people believe that if a little bit of a nutrient is good for you, then a lot must be better. This is not true. In fact, high doses of some nutrients can be harmful. Doctors might prescribe a vitamin and/or mineral supplement for people with certain health problems such as osteoporosis, anemia, or during pregnancy. Be sure to discuss vitamin and mineral supplement use with your doctor.

Nutritious Snacks

During cancer treatment your body often needs extra calories and protein to help you maintain your weight and recover and heal as quickly as possible. Nutritious snacks can help you meet those needs, maintain your strength and energy level, and enhance your feeling of well-being. To make it easier to add snacks to your daily routine, consider the following:

- Try to eat small, nutritious snacks throughout the day.
- Try to keep a variety of protein-rich snacks on hand that are easy to prepare and eat. These include yogurt, cereal and milk, half a sandwich, a bowl of hearty soup, and cheese and crackers.
- Avoid snacks that might make any treatment-related side effects worse. If you suffer from diarrhea, for example, avoid popcorn and raw fruits and vegetables. If you have a sore throat, avoid dry, coarse snacks and acidic foods.

One year of chemo left me tired and feeling "icky"—but I still carried on my regular life most of the time.

Emotional Side Effects of Breast Cancer Treatments

It is important that your focus on tests and treatments does not prevent you from considering your emotional, psychological, and spiritual health as well.

Stress: Stress is a natural part of living—working, child care, worrying about money and relationships all can cause us to feel stressed. Normal levels of stress can motivate us to take action and make changes—but when stress reaches a higher level it can cause us to feel overwhelmed and out of control. A cancer diagnosis can lead to other stressful physical changes such as tightness in your chest, throat, or face; shallow breathing; clenched fists or mouth; rapid heartbeat; sleep disturbance; and unfocused thinking. Learning or remembering ways to reduce this "distress" and finding a sense of control can make a big difference in how you manage through treatments and beyond. For example, you can learn to slow racing thoughts by changing your breathing from shallow to slow and deep breathing from the bottom of your diaphragm. Visualizing yourself in a restful or natural setting; reliving a time when you felt confident, strong, and healthy; or learning muscle relaxation techniques can all help regain a sense of control and peace.

Body image: A woman's choice of treatment will likely be influenced by her age, the image she has of herself and her body, as well as her hopes and fears. For example, some women select breast-conserving surgery with radiation therapy over a mastectomy for cosmetic and body image reasons, while others choose mastectomy because they want the affected area removed, regardless of the effect on their body image. They might be more concerned about the effects of radiation therapy and the fear of cancer returning locally than body image.

Other issues that women worry about include hair loss from chemotherapy and skin changes to the breast caused by radiation therapy. In addition to these body changes, women might also be dealing with concerns about the outcome of their treatment. These are all genuine concerns that affect how a woman makes decisions about her treatment, how she views herself, and how she feels about her treatment.

Sexuality: Concerns about sexuality are often very worrisome to a woman with breast cancer. Several factors can place a woman at higher risk for sexual problems after breast cancer. It is important to remember that some treatments for breast cancer, such as chemotherapy, can change a woman's hormone levels and may negatively affect sexual interest and/or response. A diagnosis of breast cancer when a woman is in her twenties or thirties is especially difficult because choosing a partner and childbearing are often very important during this period.

Relationship issues are also important because the diagnosis can be very distressing for the partner, as well as the patient. Partners are usually concerned about how to express their love physically and emotionally after treatment, especially surgery.

Suggestions that might help a woman adjust to changes in her body image include looking at and touching herself; seeking the support of others, preferably before surgery; involving her partner as soon as possible after surgery; and openly communicating feelings, needs, and wants created by her changed image.

Sexual impact of surgery and radiation: Because breast cancer is the most common cancer in women (excluding skin cancer), sexual problems have been linked to mastectomy more often than to any other cancer treatment. Losing a breast, or occasionally both breasts if a woman later has a second tumor, can be traumatic.

The most common sexual side effects stem from damage to a woman's feelings of attractiveness. In our culture, we are taught to view breasts as a basic part of beauty and femininity. If her breast has been removed, a woman may be insecure about whether her partner will accept her and find her sexually pleasing.

The breasts and nipples are also sources of sexual pleasure for many women. Touching the breasts is a common part of foreplay in our culture. A few women can reach orgasm just from the stroking of their breasts. For many others, breast stimulation adds to sexual excitement.

Breast surgery or radiation to the breasts does not physically decrease a woman's sexual desire, nor does it cause a "dry" vagina, lessen normal genital feelings, or make her unable to reach orgasm. Some good news from recent research is that within a year after their surgery, most women with early stage breast cancer have good emotional adjustment and sexual satisfaction. They report a quality of life similar to women who have never had cancer.

Treatment for breast cancer can interfere with pleasure from breast caressing. After a mastectomy, the whole breast is gone. Some women still enjoy being stroked around the area of the healed scar. Others dislike being touched there and might no longer even enjoy being touched on the remaining breast and nipple.

Some women who have had a mastectomy feel self-conscious being the partner "on top" during sex. The area of the missing breast is more visible in that position.

A few women have chronic pain in their chests and shoulders after radical mastectomy. During intercourse, supporting these areas with pillows may help. Also, avoid positions in which your weight rests on your chest or arms.

If surgery removed only the tumor (segmental mastectomy or lumpectomy) and was followed by radiation therapy, the breast could still be scarred, and could also be a different shape or size. During radiation therapy, the skin can become red and swollen, and the breast a little tender. Breast and nipple feeling, however, should remain normal.

Sexual impact of chemotherapy: Chemotherapy treatments can cause fatigue, nausea, and vomiting, which decrease interest in sex. Occasionally sores can occur in the vagina. After completion of chemotherapy, interest in sex gradually returns to normal.

Sexual impact of breast reconstruction: Breast reconstruction restores the shape of the breast but it cannot restore normal breast sensation. The nerve that supplies feeling to the nipple runs through the deep breast tissue, and it gets disconnected during surgery. In a reconstructed breast, the feeling of pleasure from touching the nipple is lost. A rebuilt nipple has much less feeling.

In time, the skin on the reconstructed breast will regain some sensitivity, but probably will not give the same kind of pleasure as before mastectomy. Breast reconstruction often makes women more comfortable with their bodies, however, and helps them feel more attractive.

Effect on your partner: Breast cancer can be a growth experience for couples under certain circumstances. The relationship may be enhanced if the partner participates in decision making and accompanies the woman to surgery and perhaps other treatments.

What Side Effects Can I Expect from the Surgery and Treatments?

Most cancer treatments will have some side effects, and they all create stress. Stress can make you irritable, tired, and depressed. Anesthesia, surgery, chemotherapy, and radiation are also frightening. They, too, can cause depression and tiredness.

Other side effects after surgery can include infection, tenderness, pain, scarring, lymphedema, and possibly reduced movement if you do not regularly exercise the affected arm. Some women experience numbness along the scar tissue, which is caused by nerves being cut or stretched during surgery. Nerves grow back slowly and might grow back in a different pattern, so the numbness could continue for a year or more after your surgery. A rare side effect of surgery is infection, but if you notice an angry redness, tenderness, or foul-smelling discharge you should get immediate attention and possibly start antibiotic treatment.

Before my operation I was frightened and felt alone, confused, and too depressed to seek advice. The pamphlets described medical procedures adequately, but didn't begin to tell me about all the little troubles I would have to face after the operation, such as the pain and how to ease it without overmedicating, how to get a coat on, the most beneficial arm

exercises, the discomfort of radiation burns. I found the best solution was
to wrap the burned area in an old soft sweatshirt. A book of practical
tips would be appreciated by a lot of women, I'm sure.

Most women experience some pain from breast surgery, usually along the incision and under the armpit. Pain is usually well managed by over-the-counter pain medications such as Tylenol or aspirin. Exercise and physiotherapy can help with tightness in the chest, arm, and shoulder area. If the lymph nodes are removed, there is also a risk of lymphedema caused by disruption in the normal lymph drainage. Radiation or later infection can increase the risk of developing lymphedema. If it occurs, lymphedema does not usually appear until nine months after surgery or radiation. To prevent lymphedema, it is important to avoid cuts, scrapes, bruises, or infection in the hand and arm after surgery and/or radiation.

Some of the steps that help to avoid lymphedema include:

- Avoid having blood drawn from or IVs inserted into the arm on the side of the lymph node surgery (the surgical arm).
- Do not allow a blood pressure cuff to be placed on the surgical arm. If you are in the hospital, tell all health care workers about your arm.
- If your arm or hand feels tight or swollen, don't ignore it. Tell your doctor immediately.
- If needed, wear a well-fitted compression sleeve.
- Wear gloves when gardening or doing other things that are likely to lead to cuts.

> After one friend realized it was a long trek from my upstairs bed-
> room to the downstairs fridge every time I wanted a cold drink,
> she arrived on my doorstep with a small fridge she'd purchased
> from a secondhand store.
>
> Knowing I'm a reader, many friends gave me books, lent me
> books, and recommended books. A writer friend discovered we
> were both fans of the author Ellen Gilchrist and came over to lend
> me her favorite Gilchrist books.
>
> —BERYL YOUNG

Try to get as much rest as possible, exercise moderately, and eat as
well as you can. Looking after yourself can help you cope with
treatment.

> *Following my mastectomy, I couldn't use my arm for a few months, and
> lived with pain for more than a year. Since then, everything has gone
> back to normal.*

CHEMOTHERAPY SIDE EFFECTS

> I have a friend who always talks movies and videos with me. She
> had an idea, and, like clockwork, before every treatment, arrived
> on my doorstep with new videos.
>
> —BERYL YOUNG

The side effects of chemotherapy depend on the type of drugs, the amount taken, and the length of treatment. Temporary side effects might include fatigue, nausea and vomiting, loss of appetite, hair loss, and mouth sores. Changes in the menstrual cycle may be temporary or permanent. Because chemotherapy can damage the blood-producing cells of the bone marrow, patients may have low blood cell counts. This can result in an increased chance of infection (due to a shortage of white blood cells), bleeding or bruising after minor cuts or injuries (due to a shortage of blood platelets), and fatigue (due to low red blood cell counts).

There are very effective remedies for many of the temporary side effects of chemotherapy. For example, there are several drugs that can prevent or reduce nausea and vomiting. Some anti-nausea drugs work better than others. Keep trying until you find one that works for you. A group of drugs called growth factors can help the patient's bone marrow recover after chemotherapy and can treat problems caused by low blood counts.

Premature menopause (not having any more menstrual periods) and infertility (not being able to become pregnant) are potential permanent complications of chemotherapy. The older a woman is when she receives chemotherapy, the more likely it is that she will become infertile or menopausal as a result. This can also lead to rapid bone loss from osteoporosis. Adriamycin (doxorubicin) can cause permanent heart damage if used for a long time or in high doses, but doctors carefully control the dose of this drug. They use echocardiograms and other heart tests in order to monitor the heart and will stop the medication at the first sign of damage.

My life was measured by chemo days. One week of the month I was guaranteed to be ill. It would take two weeks to recover and finally one week of feeling well before it all began again. I thank God for my fam-

ily and friends, who helped me through this trip to hell. With my chemo
days behind me, I can show all the people in my life how much I truly
love them.

Forgetfulness, Mood Swings (a.k.a. "Chemo brain")

A new friend, a former tenant, brought special English crackers for nau-
sea. We squeezed in a game of gin rummy when I was well enough,
though I credited her victories to my chemo brain.

Many women find that chemotherapy seems to make them feel depressed and forgetful, or causes dramatic mood swings. These changes are usually temporary but can often last as long as two years after chemo. Studies point to the fact that regular exercise can help. It was once thought that patients should limit physical activity during treatment, but recent research shows that maintaining (or starting) an exercise routine can help your sense of wellness and well-being during treatment. Moderate exercise helps your immune system recover its strength, and can help with the depression or mood swings that often accompany chemo.

Another side effect of chemotherapy is "chemo brain." Many women who have received chemotherapy for breast cancer will experience a slight decrease in mental functioning. There might be some difficulty in concentration and memory. This could last a long time but it rarely interferes with a woman's ability to do intellectual tasks.

It might help to talk with a friend, family member, counselor, or another woman living with breast cancer. The moods and sense of fogginess that accompany cancer treatment are a common topic at support groups, and it might help you to manage these side effects if you can talk to another patient.

> A few years ago, I'd helped a friend through lung cancer. Now she arranged for me to have massages from her own therapist. One for each of my treatments; eight massages!
>
> —BERYL YOUNG

Many cancer patients find comfort and spiritual support by focusing attention on the important relationships between themselves and their family, friends, co-workers, church, and community.

CANCER AND DEPRESSION

It is normal to grieve over the changes that cancer brings to your life. The future, which seemed so sure before, might appear to feel uncertain. Some dreams and plans can seem permanently lost as a result of a cancer diagnosis. But when you are experiencing long-lasting sadness or are having difficulty carrying out day-to-day activities, you could have clinical depression. In fact, clinical depression occurs in about 25 percent of people with cancer, causing great distress, impaired functioning, and lessens your ability to follow a treatment schedule. The good news is clinical depression is treatable.

If you have symptoms of clinical depression, you should get help. There are a number of treatments for this disorder, including medication, counseling, or a combination of both. These therapies can improve the quality of life and reduce the suffering of people with cancer.

Symptoms of Clinical Depression

- ◆ persistent sad or "empty" mood for most of the day
- ◆ loss of interest or pleasure in almost all activities for most of the day

- significant weight loss (when not dieting) or weight gain
- being "slowed down" or restless and agitated almost every day, enough for others to notice
- fatigue or loss of energy
- difficulty sleeping with early waking, sleeping too much, or not being able to sleep
- trouble concentrating, remembering, making decisions
- feelings of guilt, worthlessness, helplessness
- frequent thoughts of death or suicide (not just fear of death), suicide plans or attempts

If five or more symptoms happen nearly every day for two weeks or longer, or are severe enough to interfere with normal activities, you should be checked for clinical depression by a qualified health or mental health professional.

What to Do for Yourself or When Caring for a Person with Clinical Depression

- Encourage the depressed person to continue treatment until symptoms improve, or to seek different treatment if there is no improvement after two or three weeks.
- Promote any form of physical activity, especially mild exercise such as daily walking.
- Help make appointments for mental health treatment, if necessary.
- Provide transportation for treatment, if necessary.
- Engage your loved one in conversation and other enjoyable activities.
- Realize that negative thinking is a symptom of depression and will disappear with treatment.

- Reassure your loved one that with time and treatment, he or she will begin to feel better.
- Keep in mind that caretakers and family members can also become depressed, in which case all the above suggestions can be helpful.

Learning to accept such generous gifts has been part of this journey for me.

Most of my family live out of town but they phoned and visited often. My seventeen-year-old granddaughter came to see me, bringing a cozy pair of flannelette pajamas, and told me my wig looked great. My grandson came to town and spent part of his birthday money to buy me an ABBA tape. My eldest son brought his one-year-old to visit as often as he could, and my daughter, who lives close by, brought her four-year-old over when I was too tired to move from the sofa. Reading stories to them was the best trick I knew to forget about myself. My athletic daughter-in-law organized a team of women to walk a marathon to raise money for breast cancer research. I was a volunteer serving cold drinks at a pit stop along the way and burst into tears when "my" team stopped at the booth.

—BERYL YOUNG

Lack of Energy

Fatigue is one of the most common side effects of chemotherapy, and can range from mild lethargy to feeling completely wiped out. Fatigue tends to be worst at the beginning and at the end of a treatment cycle.

Like most other side effects, fatigue will disappear once chemotherapy is complete.

Techniques to help with fatigue include:

- Get plenty of rest and allow time during the day for periods of rest.
- Talk with your doctor or nurse about a program of regular exercise.
- Eat a well-balanced diet and drink plenty of liquids.
- Limit your activities: do only the things that are most important to you.
- Get help when you need it. Ask family, friends, and neighbors to pitch in with activities such as child care, shopping, housework, or driving. For example, neighbors might pick up some items for you at the grocery store while doing their own shopping.
- Get up slowly to help prevent dizziness when sitting or lying down.

Because chemotherapy affects the red blood cells, which contain hemoglobin and iron, some women experience anemia. Anemia can cause dizziness, shortness of breath, or chills—if you experience these symptoms, your doctor can recommend treatment.

Weight Gain

If I have to have cancer, why can't I have the good kind—the kind that makes me skinny!!!

Many women put on a few extra pounds during and after chemotherapy. This weight can be the result of a combination of hormonal changes and a reduction in physical activity levels, or a side effect of steroids that sometimes accompany treatment. Some women eat more to get rid of low-level nausea. Again, adopting a good physical fitness routine can offset this side effect. Studies have shown that even simply walking regularly can improve energy levels, and assist in weight control.

Changes in Menstrual Cycle

If you menstruate, your periods will likely become irregular or might stop altogether. For many women, periods return when their treatment is over. For some who have not yet gone through menopause, chemotherapy can cause the ovaries to stop producing estrogen and lead to early menopause.

Mouth Sores

Some people develop mouth sores during chemotherapy. Rinse your mouth with a solution of baking soda and water often during the day to clean and refresh your mouth. Drink eight to ten glasses of water and choose foods that are easy to swallow. For this side effect, and others such as diarrhea, you might want to speak to a nutritionist or members of a support group.

Taste Changes

Many people find that food doesn't taste the same during treatments. Meat especially can have a bitter or metallic taste. Choosing chicken, turkey, or fish, and using plastic utensils can help. Also limit caffeine intake.

Hygiene

Women have found it helpful to pay extra attention to hygiene and allow plenty of time to rest and recuperate in order to decrease the chances of additional sickness or infection.

Hair Loss

One of the greatest fears about chemotherapy is losing your hair—it's the most public symbol of having cancer. But hair *always* grows back after treatment ends. Also, women generally don't lose the hair under their arms or in the pubic area. Whether or not hair loss occurs depends on the particular drugs you will be receiving. Some drugs never cause hair loss while others always do. Others have different effects on the hair. Some women believe that losing hair will strip away their femininity. Hair loss might make you feel vulnerable and exposed about a very private and deeply personal matter.

Hair loss results from chemotherapy drugs slowing down the growth of the rapidly dividing cells at the roots of your hair. Your hair can become thin or you could lose it suddenly. It might come out in clumps. Frequently, it will happen about three to four weeks after your first treatment.

Some women choose to wear scarves or turbans; others buy wigs. It is important to be fitted for your wig so that it looks good on you and doesn't fall off. Don't send someone else out to buy it. If possible, choose a wig ahead of time so that the fitter can see what you look like with hair, or bring a picture of yourself to the fitting. Some women have their hair cut very short just before starting chemotherapy. If you do this, keep some of your hair for fitters to use as bangs for a turban. This sometimes helps women to adjust to hair loss.

When undergoing treatment, some women have found information provided by the Look Good, Feel Better Program to be helpful. See the Resources section at the back of this book for information about how to find the program in your area.

The impact of my diagnosis has been great on my life and the life of my family members. It's hard having the surgery, chemo, and radiation, and watching your family and friends trying to deal with it. They worry about me constantly and I hate to be a burden, although I know they don't think of me that way. One day you are going along in life and the next you're dealing with a life-threatening disease. You live with the fear of recurrence. Thank God I continue to be active in my life. I can't allow this disease to rule my life.

The end of chemotherapy can also be a difficult time for some women. Did it work? Is all the cancer gone? You no longer have the regular visits to the hospital or treatment center. You might wonder, "Is my body working for me now?" The answer is yes, but it will take time to adjust. You might not feel like yourself again for a few months. You will gradually regain your energy. If you were experiencing depression, this will lift. Your hair will grow back. You will shed the bloating and your complexion will return to normal. If you were experiencing memory loss, this will probably change (for the better!). Food will taste right again. You'll find you now crave foods you could never eat before. You are yourself again, but changed.

Since my treatment ended, I've learned to enjoy myself and to think of myself. For the first time in my life I'm also spending my money on myself. Before, I thought of my family and spouse first—no more Mrs. Nice Guy.

RADIATION SIDE EFFECTS

Radiation treatments, used as a local treatment after a lumpectomy or mastectomy, are usually given every day for three to six weeks, although this will vary from center to center.

My radiologist recommended that I go back to work immediately after treatments. My work is very stressful. I said he could go do it, but I'm taking care of me first.

Daily trips to the hospital or cancer center can be tiring and stressful. Radiation itself drains the body's energy, leaving you feeling generally weak and tired. The skin around the area receiving radiation can begin to look tanned or sunburned. It might even peel as a result of the burn, or become very dry or very moist. Your breast might be tender and aching. A light dusting of unscented cornstarch (not baby powder) will help reduce itching and will not damage the ink or tattoo marks from radiation treatment. If your skin is red, blistered, or peeling, aloe creams or cortisone creams can help. If you did not have a mastectomy, the nipple area can remain irritated or crusty for several months after treatment and this usually responds to a gentle moisture cream.

You might find that a soft, old, supportive bra, which is not tight, or a loose camisole or T-shirt is most comfortable (not wearing a bra can increase the pain and discomfort). If you did not have a mastectomy, you might notice that your treated breast has changed and become firmer than before. It usually takes about a year after radiation is over for your breast to feel and look normal again. For some woman, these changes can last longer and should be checked by you and your doctor. Some women also experience lymphedema as a result of surgery or radiation to the lymph nodes.

Other, less common effects of radiation can include inflammation in the lungs or throat, causing a dry scratchy throat or cough or a lumpy sensation in your throat.

You might feel as if you are on an emotional roller coaster as you go through the daily reminder at the clinic that you have cancer. The treatments and the anxiety can cause fatigue, fear, and weepy periods of frustration. Knowing these emotions are part of the journey through "cancer land," learning to talk to your team members about these feelings, knowing they will soon pass—all help regain your sense of control.

It's been five months since I learned I had breast cancer and I am still in radiation therapy. It's taking too long. When it started, I felt strong and confident. Now I am depressed and resentful.

HORMONE TREATMENT

Hormone treatments, like tamoxifen (Nolvadex), are used to treat tumors that are sensitive to hormones. Tamoxifen stops estrogen from binding to the breast cells. This stops or slows the growth of cancerous cells, which depend on estrogen for growth. Tamoxifen is administered as a pill, taken daily. Side effects can include hot flashes, mood swings, vaginal dryness, changes in vision, and nausea for the first month. Tamoxifen use has been linked to endometrial cancer and blood clots in rare cases. There is now good evidence that the optimal duration for tamoxifen treatment is five years. You and your doctor should monitor the effects throughout your treatment.

You may also want to discuss the newer kinds of hormone treatment drugs, called aromatase inhibitors, that are now being used in the treatment of early stage breast cancer. There are three aromatase inhibitors: anastrozole (Arimidex), femora (Letrozole), and exemestane (Aromasin). They are not linked to blood clots and endometrial cancer but can cause osteoporosis.

The side effects of tamoxifen are a pain to deal with. However, in the final analysis, they are a small price to pay. I am healthy, disease free, and very much alive.

Looking After Yourself During Treatment

Things you can learn from a dog:

- ◆ Never pass up the opportunity for a joyride.
- ◆ Allow the experience of fresh air and wind in your face to be pure ecstasy.
- ◆ When the loved ones come home, run to greet them.
- ◆ When it's in your best interest, practice obedience.
- ◆ Take naps and stretch before rising.
- ◆ Romp and play daily.
- ◆ Eat with gusto.
- ◆ Be loyal.
- ◆ Never pretend to be something that you're not.
- ◆ If you want what lies buried, dig until you find it.
- ◆ When someone is having a bad day, be silent, sit close by, and nuzzle them gently.
- ◆ Thrive on attention and let people touch you.
- ◆ Avoid biting when a simple growl will do.
- ◆ On hot days, drink lots of water and lie under a shady tree.
- ◆ When you're happy, dance around and wag your whole body.
- ◆ Bond with your pack.
- ◆ Delight in the simple joys of a long walk.

—PATTY WOOTEN,
registered nurse, reprinted from
Jest for the Health of It

Things to Consider During and After Treatment

During and after your treatment for breast cancer you might be able to speed up your recovery and improve your quality of life by taking an active role. Learn about the benefits and risks of each of your treatment options, and ask questions of your cancer care team if there is anything you do not understand. Learn about and look out for side effects of treatment, and report these right away to your cancer care team so they can take steps to ease them.

Remember that your body is as unique as your personality and your fingerprints. Although understanding your cancer's stage and learning about your treatment options can help predict what health problems you could face, no one can say for sure how you will respond to cancer or its treatment.

You might have special strengths, such as a history of excellent nutrition and physical activity, a strong family support system, or a deep faith, and these strengths may make a difference in how you respond to cancer. There are also experienced professionals in mental health services, social work services, and pastoral services who may assist you in coping with your illness.

You can also help in your own recovery from cancer by making healthy lifestyle choices. If you use tobacco, stop now. Quitting will improve your overall health, and the full return of the sense of smell may help you enjoy a healthy diet during recovery. If you use alcohol, limit the amount you drink. Have no more than one drink per day. Good nutrition can help you get better after treatment. Eat a nutritious and balanced diet, with plenty of fruits, vegetables, and whole-grain foods.

If you are being treated for cancer, be aware of the battle that is going on in your body. Radiation therapy and chemotherapy add to the fatigue caused by the disease itself. To help you with the fatigue, plan your daily activities around when you feel your best. If you can, get plenty of sleep at night. And ask your cancer care team about a daily exercise program to help you feel better.

SUMMARY

A cancer diagnosis and treatment are a major life challenge that impacts not only you but everyone who cares for you. Although it requires stamina, energy, and commitment, your ability and willingness to actively participate in decision making and treatment can help reduce fear and confusion. Before you get to the point where you feel overwhelmed, consider talking with someone trained in helping manage the emotional and psychological challenges of dealing with cancer. You might also consider attending a meeting of a local support group. If you need assistance in other ways, contact your hospital's social service department or the American Cancer Society or Canadian Cancer Society, which will help you find resources in your area.

One fall day, an old friend arrived to give me a day's clean-up work in my patio garden. Then, when Christmas was coming and I was overwhelmed at the thought of it, another friend took me shopping; still another came over to wrap the presents I'd bought for my family. Out-of-town friends helped too. A Web-savvy pal offered to be my "information source." I'd e-mail her questions about treatments and back would come the answers that saved me hours of frustration.

—BERYL YOUNG

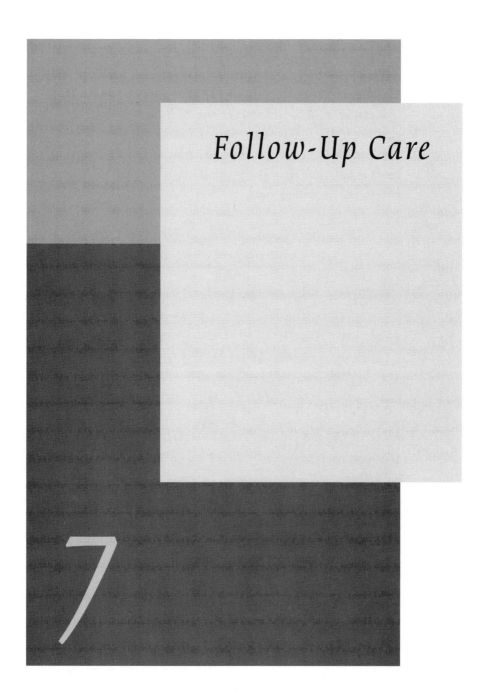

Follow-Up Care

7

This chapter is about the emotional and practical realities of getting on with life after your treatments are over. It also provides information about the different kinds of surgery and implants that can be used to reconstruct breast tissue. Not all women choose to have breast reconstruction and many find they are comfortable with one breast or no breast. These choices can be made at any time from the point of diagnosis until years and years after treatment ends.

> *What I found to be of huge benefit was the ability to meet with a nurse and doctor twice a year, people who were really focused on my health.*

> *Sleeping Beauty was awakened by Prince Charming. It took cancer for me to step out of my lethargy. My priorities changed. I realized the urgency and importance of taking my life into my own hands, to live according to my desires, to go and get what I need, and not to accept what I do not want to. Cancer has given me a taste for life—a passionate one.*

What to Expect After Your Treatment Ends

Your follow-up care will depend on the type of treatment you have had and the region you live in. Usually, after your chemotherapy or radiation is over, or after surgery and recovery, you will see your family doctor, surgeon and/or oncologist(s) every three to twelve months for the first two years. After two years, you will probably have appointments once every four to twelve months for the following three years. After that, you should have an annual checkup with your family doctor. Your doctor should ask how you are coping and about any physical changes. S/he will probably order blood tests and a mammogram and do a breast exam. Some doctors will order a chest X-ray. You should also see your family doctor for a regular Pap test, pelvic exam and periodic testing for colon cancer.

If you have not already been shown how to do a breast self-examination (BSE), ask your doctor to show you how or to refer you to someone who can. You might also want to show your doctor how you do BSE to make sure you are doing it right, especially because of the changes your body has been through. Also, learn to examine your scar tissue for any changes.

You should also have a mammogram on an annual basis. Women who have already had breast cancer are three to four times more likely to develop a new tumor (in the same breast or the other one) as women who've never had the disease. They are also at risk of having their cancer return in the same breast if they didn't have a mastectomy. Regular mammograms can help find recurrences or new cancers at an early stage, when they are easier to treat. If possible, you should have your mammogram done at the same clinic or hospital each time, or ask that your previous mammograms be transferred so they are available for comparison. If you had a breast reconstruction with implants, tell the technologist doing the mammogram. Ask if they are experienced doing imaging (X-rays) on implanted breasts.

Some women aren't emotionally prepared for how difficult their annual checkup can be. The uncertainty of whether or not your cancer has come back can be very distressing. It might be helpful to talk to someone who has already been through this. Bring along someone you trust to these appointments if it will make you feel more comfortable and reassured.

Except for the fear of recurrence, especially around mammography time, the quality of my life is the same as it was, maybe even better.

You might still feel sad after treatment ends. The sadness can be due to a sense of grief or loss, especially if you had a mastectomy. We all grieve in different ways and at our own pace. The sadness, the crying, and the depression will eventually be replaced by a fierce hope and the newfound joy in such simple things as a sunrise or the company of a good friend.

> *Losses were small in terms of transient discomfort and appearance. Many gains were learning to live more fully and openly. I have a better quality of life now—no time for pettiness, gossip, complainers. I am content with what I have and enjoy life to the fullest. I do everything I want to do.*

Breast Reconstruction and Prosthesis

Today, many women's treatment involves breast-conserving surgery such as lumpectomy. This means that most of the breast is saved. However, if you had a mastectomy, you may want to consider breast reconstruction.

An estimated two million American women and half a million Canadian women have been through breast cancer treatment. Society is starting to adjust to our one-breasted presence! Still, for other women, replacing their lost breast is worth the discomfort of facing another surgery. Approximately 20 percent of women who have mastectomy surgery will choose to have reconstruction. Some women will have reconstructive surgery at the same time or very soon after a mastectomy. Others will wait for many years before they decide. The choice is up to you.

> *I was only thirty-five when I lost my breast. After becoming an activist, I saw my mastectomy scar as a badge of courage—the mark of the*

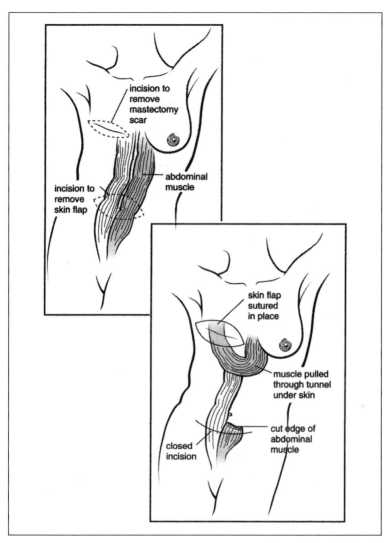

FIGURE 7.1 *Reconstruction using your own tissue involves moving living muscle from the lower abdomen to the area of the mastectomy scar.*

Amazon warrior that I had become. I spent ten years working as an advocate in Canada and the U.S. in the late 1980s and through the 1990s when breast cancer wasn't trendy and we had to be brave pioneers. My daughters were so little when I was diagnosed that they didn't know me any other way. When they got older, they would ask me to change where no one could see me at the YMCA pool. As I grew older, I grew tired of always being a warrior. After the reconstruction, everyone wanted to know, "How come now and not before?" I couldn't say why, but the time had come for me to be a plain old, smart, sexy woman—just like everyone else.

In the past decade, the methods for breast reconstruction have greatly improved. Although a reconstructed breast will never look or feel exactly like your original breast, nor ever be able to make milk or have a nipple that becomes erect, the results can be very good.

There are two types of breast reconstruction. One involves using implants; the other uses pieces of the woman's own tissue (sometimes called "flaps") from elsewhere on her body. There are risks associated with each type.

BREAST IMPLANTS

Breast implants are made of a silicone shell that contains a sterile water-based solution. The implant is placed behind the muscle or breast tissue; therefore it does not make it harder to discover another lump, should the cancer return. You will be able to do breast self-examination and have a mammogram.

The risks of having a surgical implant are the possibility that the scar will become infected or that the implant will fail; that is, it might become hard or the tissue over it could shrink. There has been some controversy in recent years about the long-term safety of silicone

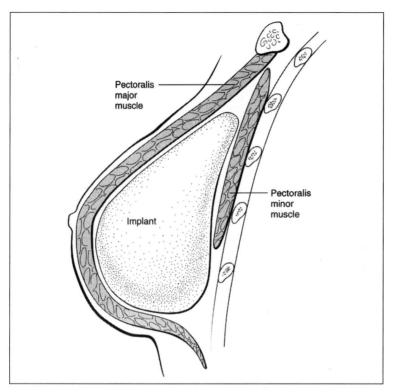

FIGURE 7.2 *Placement of the internal silicone implant under the chest*

breast implants. If you would like to read more about this, see the Resources section at the end of the book.

> *I do not dwell on the diagnosis. At times there is an overwhelming feeling of "why me?". But having the implants made all the difference to me.*

BREAST RECONSTRUCTION

If you want breast reconstruction, discuss it with your surgeon and oncologist before your first surgery. It is important to remember that breast reconstruction is major surgery. It is better to have the reconstruction after completing radiation or chemotherapy so it doesn't interfere with your treatment. It may be possible for your surgeon and plastic surgeon to do both procedures at the same time, but they are usually done separately. Having radiation may have an effect on the elasticity of your skin and therefore the type (and the size!) of the reconstruction, so it's better to talk with a plastic surgeon early on, especially if you are strongly committed to reconstruction. Breast reconstruction is almost always possible after mastectomy. In both the U.S. and Canada, it is fully covered by health insurance plans.

> *Reconstruction has been one of the great joys of my life. I really feel that my recovery didn't truly begin until I had reconstruction. I marvel at the "magic of science" and feel blessed to have had access to the best and most talented specialists in this field. My only regret is that I didn't have a bilateral!*

HOW DO I BUY A PROSTHESIS?

Many women, who have had a mastectomy, will choose to wear a breast prosthesis. In the early recovery period after your surgery, it is best to wear a lightweight prosthesis to avoid putting any pressure on the scar and surrounding tissue. The prothesis is usually made of fabric or foam and covered with a light, stretchy material. Once your healing is further along, you can choose a more permanent breast form. Prostheses are made to be comfortable and look and feel natural. If you can, speak with someone who has already been through this process to recommend a good prosthesis fitter in your area. She might also be able to offer you advice on when to buy your prosthesis.

> *I used a prosthesis in my bra for three years, but then decided to remake the breast with the use of abdominal muscle. I am happy.*

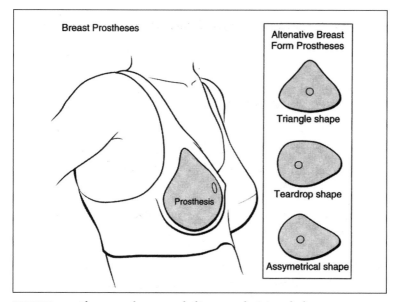

FIGURE 7.3   *Placement of an external silicone prosthesis into the bra*

Usually, your scar is healed enough after a few weeks to wear a prosthesis, which you can buy from a mastectomy boutique or prosthesis fitter. Look in the Resources section at the end of this book or under "Breast Prosthesis" in the telephone directory, or ask the local unit of the American Cancer Society or Canadian Cancer Society. Most fitters require an appointment, which will take about an hour. You might want to ask your husband, partner, or a friend to come with you to the appointment.

> We have come a long way in twenty-seven years! When I had cancer I
> had nobody to talk to. I lost both my breasts and my ovaries in one year.
> My two boys were four and six years old. We had just moved into our
> house and money was tight. I made my prosthesis from an old bra filled
> with birdseed and sand. For more than twenty years I have been a

volunteer with the Reach for Recovery program and have learned a lot
from the couple of hundred women I have seen. All are different.

Permanent prostheses are more realistic and can be made of polyester, foam rubber, or a soft fleshlike material containing liquid or silicone gel. A prosthesis is designed to weigh the same as normal breast tissue, so when you wear it you won't feel lopsided or experience back and shoulder pain. The prosthesis might seem heavy at first and can take some getting used to. It will also warm to your body temperature even though it might feel cold at first.

Mastectomy boutiques also sell bras with a pocket of fabric to hold your prosthesis in place, as well as bathing suits with a bra lining that has a prosthesis pocket. A properly fitted prosthesis should not move around, rub, or irritate your skin. Once in place, you should be able to forget it is there. If you have problems or feel discomfort, go back to your fitter for an adjustment or replacement.

Group or private insurance plans might cover the cost of the prosthesis. Check with your local breast cancer support group, private or government health insurance plan, or the cancer society in your area. In most cases, a breast prosthesis that is covered by insurance can be replaced every two years if needed.

ADJUSTING TO YOUR NEW BODY
Some women decide not to undergo reconstruction or wear prosthesis. Every woman has a different sense of self and of personal identity, and there is no right answer—just what you're comfortable with.

After having a bilateral mastectomy at thirty-nine, I thought for sure
I'd have reconstruction. But six months out, the idea of another major
surgery, added to the fact that I'd only end up with an A cup anyway
because I'd had previous radiation, changed my mind. I find my pros-

thesis uncomfortable, so mostly I just go without. My partner thinks I
look aerodynamic.

Menopausal Symptoms and Breast Cancer

There are a number of different reasons your body goes into menopause with breast cancer treatment.

Certain chemotherapy drugs bring about early menopause by knocking out ovarian function—this is called medical menopause. For example, half of women aged thirty-five or younger and about 80 percent of those aged thirty-five to forty-four who take CMF (combination chemotherapy drugs cyclphosphamide, methotrexate, and hudrouralil), go into menopause. The risk of permanent menopause is less with adriamycin chemotherapy (AC). Occasionally, chemo-induced menopause is temporary. Premenopausal women, who've been rendered post-menopausal by treatment, run a high risk of early bone loss, so it's a good idea to get a baseline bone density test as early as you can, monitor the situation carefully, and then consider having annual tests. There are lots of ways bone loss can be minimized and averted if it's addressed early, including weight-bearing exercise, diet, and drugs. It is a good idea to take vitamin D and calcium supplements.

Surgical removal of your ovaries (oophorectomy), which is sometimes done in premenopausal ER-positive women, instantly induces menopause.

The hot flashes sometimes associated with menopause are also side effects of tamoxifen and other anti-estrogen adjuvant therapies. While these drugs don't cause menopause *per se*, their side effect can mimic the symptoms.

Going off hormone replacement therapy, which most doctors recommend upon breast cancer diagnosis, can induce menopause. You might experience a combined natural/medical menopause that is the result of a sudden drop in estrogen levels.

SYMPTOM RELIEF

Several treatments have been studied and found to relieve menopausal symptoms:

- *Hot flashes:* Venlafaxine, a relatively new antidepressant medication marketed as Effexor. If this does not work then gabapentin may help
- *Vaginal dryness:* K-Y lubricating jelly and Replens, a vaginal moisturizer
- *Sexual and urinary problems:* Estradiol vaginal rings such as Estring, which provide controlled local delivery of very low doses of estrogen (creams are *not* recommended because the estrogen in them passes into the blood, and this can lead to high concentrations of estrogen in the body). Recently a vaginal suppository (Vagifem) that releases low doses of estrogen into the vagina has been used. However, if used frequently it can lead to high concentrations of estrogen in the body.

Other treatments have been found to improve bone mass and reduce the risk of osteoporosis:

- Exercise, a diet rich in calcium, and appropriate mineral and vitamin supplements
- Bone-strengthening drugs called bisphosphonates
- Alternative treatments include acupuncture, various hormone preparations, herbs, and vitamins; however, there is not sufficient evidence to determine effectiveness.

One drug used to treat osteoporosis that is *not* recommended for women who have had breast cancer is raloxifene, a selective estrogen receptor modulator. Although it is similar to tamoxifen, a drug commonly used in the treatment of breast cancer, there are no studies supporting raloxifene's use by women with breast cancer.

Pregnancy After Breast Cancer

Because of the well-established link between estrogen levels and the growth of breast cancer cells, many doctors have advised breast cancer survivors not to become pregnant for at least two years after treatment. This pause would allow any early return of the cancer to be diagnosed and could affect a woman's decision to become pregnant. But two years is an arbitrary number and earlier pregnancy might not be harmful. After breast cancer, endocrine therapy (tamoxifen or aromatase inhibitor) is given for approximately five years. If a woman is contemplating pregnancy, she should be aware that endocrine therapy, which is given to prevent breast cancer recurrence, will be interrupted.

Of the few studies that have been conducted, nearly all have found that pregnancy does not increase the risk of recurrence after successful treatment of breast cancer. Women are advised to discuss their risk of recurrence with their doctors. In some cases, counseling can help women with the complex issues and uncertainties regarding motherhood and breast cancer survivorship.

Hormone Replacement Therapy after Breast Cancer

The known link between estrogen levels and breast cancer growth has discouraged many women and their doctors from choosing or recommending hormone replacement therapy (HRT). Unfortunately, many women experience menopausal symptoms after treatment for breast cancer. This can occur naturally or develop as a result of menopausal women stopping HRT. Chemotherapy can also cause early menopause in premenopausal women.

In the past, doctors have offered HRT after breast cancer treatment to women suffering from severe menopausal symptoms because early studies had shown no harm. However, in early 2004, the HABITS study found that breast cancer survivors taking HRT were much more likely to develop a new or recurrent breast cancer than women who were not taking the drugs. For this reason, most doctors now feel that for women previously treated for breast cancer, taking HRT would be unwise.

Women should consider discussing with their doctors alternatives to HRT pills to help with specific menopausal symptoms. Some doctors have suggested that phytoestrogens (estrogen-like substances from certain plant sources such as soy products) might be safer than the estrogens used in HRT. However, there is not enough information available on phytoestrogens to evaluate their safety for breast cancer survivors.

SUMMARY

Your time after treatment will not make you forget the cancer or the thought that it might recur. Cancer might have robbed you of a belief of your own immortality. But surviving the crisis can also be a gift: learning to live in the moment, appreciating each day.

By the end of my treatment we would ride for half an hour, a simple loop through the neighborhood...about halfway through the ride we reached a short steep hill. I thought I was keeping up, but the truth was, my friends were being kind. In fact, they were moving so slowly they almost fell over sideways on their bikes...I had little concept of how fast or how slow we were moving.

All of a sudden, a figure moved up on my left. It was a woman in her 50s on a heavy mountain bike, and she went right by me.

—LANCE ARMSTRONG, *It's Not about the Bike*

Learning More about the Impact of Cancer on Families, Friends, Intimacy, and Relationships

8

When a woman is diagnosed with breast cancer, her husband, lover, partner, close friends, and family members can help contribute in many ways to her emotional healing. This chapter is for you and the people who are close to you to read together and learn about how to help each other through this experience.

After eighteen years of marriage, I'd been separated for two months and was fresh off a double mastectomy. I met my new partner, also a cancer survivor, while doing a spinning fundraiser on the survivor bike. Even though I had lifted my shirt many, many times for curious women, I was uncomfortable revealing anything to him. I thought I would get more comfortable after the exchange from the tissue expanders to the implants, but I didn't—I still hid them behind a bra. Six months into our relationship we were bicycling together on a four-day cycling fundraiser. It was the first day of the ride and the facilities that we used for our showers was an arena. There was a huge lineup for the showers. It obviously was going to be quicker if we just went in and showered together. So we did. He teased me that he wouldn't look. At that moment it suddenly hit me that he really didn't care what my boobs looked like. After that day, I was fine about him seeing them, but there is no touching involved. I am not sure if that will ever change. I just got my nipples done a couple of weeks ago and will be going for the tattoos in six weeks. At least they will look sort of normal. Just a lot of scars. But that's fine with me.

Staying Connected

Like other serious illnesses, cancer can bring couples closer but it can also magnify existing tensions in your relationship. Learning how to talk and listen to one another—without being defensive or judgmen-

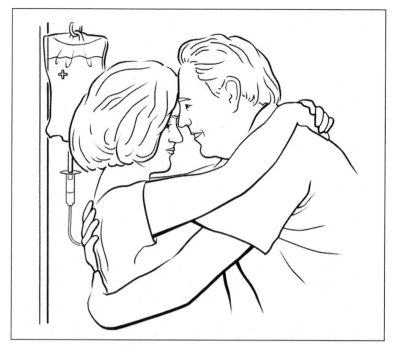

FIGURE 8.1   *Intimacy after breast cancer*

tal—can help your relationship to survive, and even grow, during this difficult time.

Whether it is your husband, your lover, or your partner, his or her experience of cancer and yours are not the same. That person is afraid of losing you, afraid that you are suffering. But they might also feel they need to be "strong," to "hold the family together."

> *It is very important to educate the husband that what a woman needs in these times is love. He should meet with the doctor to really know what his wife is going through.*

Both of you are trying to understand the complex issues of treatment and diagnosis while simultaneously dealing with your own reactions and emotions. There are ways you can learn to cope with your feelings and still provide emotional and practical help for each other. You can cope by:

- Going together to the doctor's appointments and asking questions
- Keeping a record of questions and the answers
- Keeping a journal of your thoughts and feelings
- Attending a support group for couples or information sessions at your cancer treatment center. Call the American Cancer Society or the Canadian Cancer Society for more information.
- Talking with other people who have had similar experiences
- Keeping up a program of regular exercise, bodywork, or tai chi
- Escaping from the intense pressure of "having cancer" by reading, listening to music, watching movies, enjoying restaurant dinners, or visiting friends
- Making plans for your future
- Trying meditation, prayer, and guided imagery

> *I left my spouse because I could not stand his indifference. I felt as though I was living by myself and felt very lonely. He never took care of me. I'm happier now.*

FOR HUSBANDS AND PARTNERS

Your wife or partner is probably struggling with feelings of fear, anger, depression, vulnerability, and a sense of being "out of control." Let her know that she can share these feelings with you, that they are not "right" or "wrong" and you want to know what she is feeling and thinking. Listen without judging her or trying to provide answers or assurances that "everything is fine." You both know cancer is not "fine"—false assurances don't help. But listening, being supportive, and helping to understand the disease and its treatments will help her regain confidence in the present and maintain hope for your future together.

> At first, my husband was great. Now he doesn't even want to talk about it. It's like he's pretending it's not happening!

Many women find they need to talk about breast cancer for a lot longer than their families and friends want to hear about it. And women fear that they will be abandoned if they are too needy, too demanding of support. One solution is to talk to other women in a support group.

> I just got married in April. I have never been married before and have no children. We were hoping there might be a chance we could have at least one. Then I find out I have cancer. It has been a heavy financial burden, and since half of my husband's wages go to child support payments, I need to work. This has added more stress. But I have a very gentle, loving, and understanding husband, who has helped me through this more than anyone. I feel your partner's attitude toward you makes a big difference in the healing process. I wouldn't be getting through this so well without my husband's love and support. He makes me feel like a whole person.

ASSUMING NEW ROLES

Because women typically have a greater share of the homemaking or caregiving responsibilities within families, we often find it difficult to suddenly find ourselves being the ones receiving care. The changing dynamic leads to a new role for partners, who can feel unprepared to assume the role of primary caregiver to a spouse with breast cancer, and thus face distress and caregiver burnout.

Breast cancer has been a gift. I have learned to say "I." I have learned to say "no." Even though I lost a breast I feel more whole than when I had both breasts.

ADJUSTING TO LIFE AFTER TREATMENT TOGETHER

Since people go through so many different phases during the course of an illness that can be as unpredictable and persistent as cancer, learning to listen without jumping in and trying to fix everything is especially important.

The period just after treatment is particularly vulnerable for couples. Many partners assume—wrongly—that things will get back to normal after treatments are over. Many women go through a transitional phase during which they are recovering from the physical and psychological impact of the illness, and may still feel very vulnerable and in need of ongoing support. This can lead to tension in a relationship when there are new or different expectations that are unspoken. Couples can work through these challenges by treating the post-treatment period as a time for transition and adjustment, adapting by setting new goals for themselves as a couple, and maintaining a sense of humor throughout.

THE NIGHTLY RITUAL
I prop my wig on the dresser,
And tuck my prosthesis beneath
And thank God I still go to bed with
My man and my very own teeth.

FERTILITY AFTER CANCER TREATMENT

Cancer treatment can leave some women infertile. If the woman is still young, the couple must grapple with grief about the inability to have a baby. Many couples have found new ways to rebuild commitment in the relationship by working on creating new plans and dreams. Couples struggling with these issues should request a referral to a therapist who is experienced in dealing with couples and illness.

I love that Ken wants to have children. But who knows what my health will allow? But whatever happens, I suppose I will always consider things like the cancer support community as my child. It's so special and like a doting parent I'm so proud of it.

Despite these challenges, a breast cancer diagnosis can bring a couple closer together. Being brought face to face with mortality often drives home the point that one day they will be separated by death, and this often strengthens their bond, sometimes uniting them even more.

—SUSAN G. KOMEN,
*"What's Happening to the Woman
I Love? Couples Coping with Breast Cancer,"
Breast Cancer Foundation, 1999.*

Practical Help

Knowing how to help can be difficult at times. Here are some tips:

- Go with her to appointments, clinic visits, and group meetings.
- Cook dinner or order out if the smell of food upsets her.
- Help keep your children occupied and cared for.
- Hire a cleaning person to keep the home tidy.
- Screen calls and let friends and family know she appreciates their concern but needs to rest.

- Make plans for quiet times (e.g., music, flowers, a warm bath with scented oils).
- Take a romantic weekend away—and remember that romance isn't just about sex.
- Keep the garden tidy and weeded.
- Help her to participate in daily activities if she wants to.
- Make an effort to sit and hold hands, without TV or kids or distractions.
- Take a walk.

Emotional Help

Here are some ways in which emotional support can be given:

- Spend time together—give her your attention and enjoy the comfortable silence of good friends.
- Ask her to explain what is helpful and what isn't.
- Allow her to express her emotions—including anger—and try not to take it personally when she takes her anger out on you. Cancer is unfair and we don't always act on our best behavior when we're sick.
- Let her know it's okay to cry and be sad, angry, or just quiet.
- Give her your love and remind her what you admire about her, what your relationship has meant, and why you are friends.
- Write a letter or poem telling her how much she means to you.
- Touch her, hold her hand, hug her, and be gentle.

Remember, you won't be able to do everything, but you *are* making a difference in the life of the woman you love and care about.

If I ever wondered what my husband's responses to a medical crisis
would be, I don't have to worry anymore: his support has been out-

standing. If a terrible event can have a positive side, it is this: we are
closer than ever.

SEX AFTER BREAST CANCER

For some women, breast cancer will bring no change in their sexual feelings. Others will find their sexuality enhanced as a result of such a life-transforming experience. Still others have a temporary lack of sexual desire because of the effects of their treatment or because they do not feel comfortable with their changed body. Some chemotherapy (and the potential side effect of early menopause in younger women) can cause vaginal dryness and pain during intercourse, and can also lead to diminished libido in the longer term. And some women may never have considered sexuality as an important part of their lives and may consider it even less so after breast cancer.

Stress, worry, anesthesia, pain, radiation and chemotherapy, feeling ill, and being tired are all powerful depressants, and any depressant is likely to reduce sexual desire. Vaginal lubricants can help with the physical issues, and good communication is extremely important; couples can work together so that intimacy remains even in the absence of the sex life they had before breast cancer.

Time and patience can be the best solutions to many sex-related issues. Generally, if sex was good before, it will be good again. "Again" frequently comes a few months after the end of your treatment, about the time that your body stops feeling like someone else's and starts to feel more like home.

> *My husband and I both had cancer surgery within six months of each*
> *other; he had his penis removed and I lost a breast. What a pair of*
> *"bookends" we made! He died three years ago of a heart attack. Our*
> *sense of humor got us that far.*

It is also true that sex has as much to do with the mind as the body—and everything to do with the heart. At first you may feel shy or fear rejection; you may need to wear your prosthesis and bra and nightgown and robe to bed. A good, kind, and patient lover loves you, not just one of your breasts. Your lover is waiting for some sort of signal from you that you're ready to make love again. That lovemaking may not set off any fireworks, but then, did you expect it to every time before? Not having a breast, or part of a breast, may mean a few changes in what you're used to doing. But then, you may discover areas of excitement you didn't suspect you had. A good time in bed isn't just for women with two all-natural breasts, or beautiful people, or young people. Good sex is for people who want it enough to make it happen.

SEXUALITY AND SINGLE WOMEN

Single women who've had breast cancer, especially those who've had partial or complete mastectomies, face unique challenges. The prospect of dating and intimacy is daunting. How do I tell this new person about my situation? It's advisable to make sure you've established a base friendship before jumping into intimacy. Your breast cancer is an intimate dimension of your character, and should probably not be disclosed until you'd consider disclosing other intimate details of your life. Sometimes, revealing this information too soon can intimidate prospective partners, so don't let breast cancer stop you from getting out into the dating world, but don't make yourself too vulnerable by assuming that you have to tell your breast cancer status until you're comfortable doing so.

How Much Should I Tell My Children or Grandchildren?

Even very young children know when something is wrong. Pretending that everything is normal only increases their fears. It is much kinder to share what you know in a way that they can understand. A very young child can be told that your breast was sick and you had to have an operation, and now you have to take medicine that makes you very tired. This gives the child a chance to help you, for example, by playing quietly while you rest. It also gives the child an opportunity to talk about his or her own fears that you are sick, and that you might go to the hospital. This kind of talking makes it easier for both mother and child to be able to admit to being frightened and uncertain.

Younger children often worry about two things:

* *Who is going to take care of me?* They need to feel safe and protected. They need to know somebody will take care of them
* *Is Mommy going to die?* Be honest with your children and don't make promises that you aren't sure you can keep. Be hopeful and realistic: "I can't say exactly what will happen to me but I'm taking medicines that can help me get better. I'm working with the doctors to get better as soon as possible."

Try to maintain some of your normal routine and create the sense of safety and caring that will help your children adjust. Tell them honestly about the changes that might happen to your appearance. Encourage them to express their feelings by drawing or singing.

Older children can be angry or withdraw. But often, when they know what the problem is and that they are safe, they feel free to talk about their fears. They could also help out around the house, which will help them feel they are contributing to your recovery.

If they don't feel comfortable talking about their fears with you, they can talk to someone else. Cancer is now so common that many children and teens are able to get information and support from friends who have experienced cancer in their own families. Your child's teachers, a school nurse, or cancer center support groups may have information about support services for children. You might find it helpful to talk to your oncologist about your children's reactions to your diagnosis. Often the oncologist can bring a member of your treatment team, such as an experienced nurse or social worker, to talk with your children about cancer.

> *My children had a lot of trouble coping with me being ill. In hindsight, they probably should have gone to a Kids Can Cope program.*

If your children are adults, they might have concerns about their own health. Daughters, in particular, might worry about their risk of developing breast cancer. Teenage daughters, for example, may express anger and resentment towards a sick mother. Share this book with them and encourage them to find out more about their own risks. Encourage your adult daughters to do breast self-examinations (BSE) and, when appropriate, to get routine mammograms. In some cities, breast cancer support groups offer support and information for adult children of people who have had cancer.

Other Big Cs

Cancer has often been called the "Big C." There are other big Cs.

+ *Control* is taking an active part in your care and survival. Control involves sorting out your priorities in life and making choices to give you the greatest possible chance of long-term survival.
+ *Compassion* for yourself, first and foremost, is essential. As women, we spend most of our time looking after others. As someone's wife, lover, mother, daughter, sister, neighbor, helper, employer, or employee, we are always serving the needs of others. Now your needs must come first.

> *I've slowed down and relaxed a lot. I no longer try to perform at the 250 percent rate. One hundred percent is now good enough for me.*

Compassion is also for the people who share your life. Although they do not have cancer, they too may be grieving because you have changed. You may not have as much time and energy for them as you did. They may be terrified of having to face a future without you.

+ *Communication* can change in your relationships. Cancer places heavy demands on relationships and strains communication. Hopefully, good relationships will stay good, and even improve. Troubled relationships might get overburdened under the crisis. Cancer doesn't cause divorce. It doesn't cause kids to leave home. But poor communication does cause additional and unnecessary suffering.

SUMMARY

When the person who has been the family nurturer suddenly becomes the one most in need of support and care, it is a big change. Roles have shifted. Unwritten rules have changed. And for families unable to talk openly and respectfully, there will be trouble and pain.

You will have to ask for the help you need. You might have to give up some basic household tasks, reduce your work hours (inside or outside your home), and say no to requests for volunteering. You will have to make caring of you your full-time job right now.

I have had a very bad five years. My husband had a bad stroke and I had to look after him. At the same time, I broke my ankle and arm— and found the lump. My main concern was looking after my husband and I worried about what would happen to him if I died. He passed away in May. I'm still going to the clinic that has been so kind to me and I love them all.

After a while, you learn the subtle difference
between holding a hand and chaining a soul.
And you learn that love doesn't mean possession
and company doesn't mean security,
and loneliness is universal.
And you learn that kisses aren't contracts,
and presents aren't promises . . .
and you begin to accept your defeats
with your head up and your eyes open,
with the grace of a woman, not the grief of a child.

And you learn to build all of your hope on today,
because tomorrow's ground is too uncertain,
and futures have a way of falling down in mid-flight
because tomorrow's ground can be too uncertain for plans;
yet each step taken in a new direction creates a path
towards the promise of a brighter dawn.
After a while you learn that even sunshine burns
if you get too much.
So you plant your own garden,
and nourish your own soul
instead of waiting for someone to bring you flowers.
And you learn that you really can endure ...
That you really are strong,
and you really do have worth.
And you learn and grow ...
With every good-bye you learn.

—VERONICA SHOFFSTALL

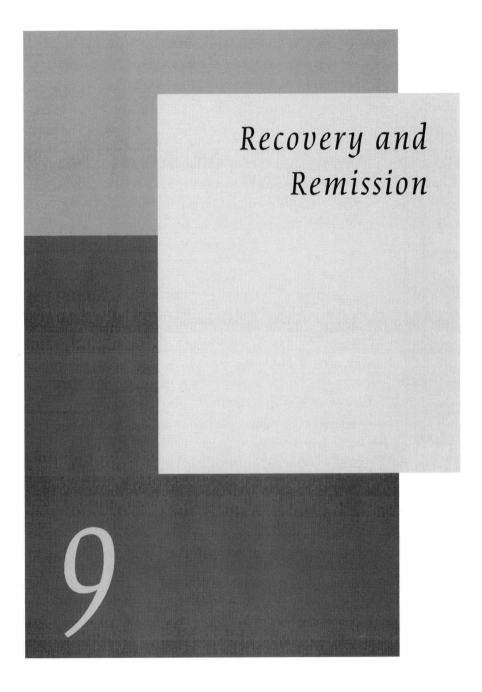

Recovery and
Remission

9

This chapter will help you understand life after treatment, including ways you can reduce the risk of your cancer returning, and adjusting to the changes that cancer can bring.

> You may in the privacy of the heart take out the album of your own life and search it for the people and places you have loved and learned from yourself, and for those moments in the past—many of them half forgotten—through which you glimpsed, however dimly and fleetingly, the sacredness of your own journey.
>
> —FREDERICK BUECHNER, *The Sacred Journey*

Life after Breast Cancer

LIVING WITH UNCERTAINTY

What Is Living with Uncertainty?

The uncertainties that cancer can cause do not always end with treatment. While the immediate illness may be in remission, you may find that your life has changed in unexpected ways. You may feel uncertain about the changes that cancer caused and worry about what your life is going to be like after cancer. Many cancer survivors find that they feel unsure about many aspects of their lives. This is called living with uncertainty.

Some things survivors may be uncertain about:

- Their health
- The quality of their medical care

- How long they will live after treatment
- Their careers

You may be able to live with uncertainty in your life and remain positive. However, living with uncertainty can also be very difficult and upsetting. Some survivors think that if they aren't certain about most things in their life, then bad things are likely to happen. It's important to realize that there are some things, like how long you are going to live, that you can't know for sure. However, it is possible to learn to live with uncertainty and not feel so overwhelmed by the things you don't know and can't control.

Do All Survivors Live with Uncertainty?

All cancer survivors live with some uncertainty about their future, but it affects different people in different ways. How you deal with it could be related more to your personality and coping style than the type of cancer or treatment you received. It could also be related to how much you think about cancer.

- You may put your cancer experience in the past and choose to hardly ever think about it. The uncertainties that cancer causes may not bother you very much.
- You may think about cancer often and find your thoughts are overwhelming. You may live with a lot of fears about whether the cancer will come back or how your cancer will affect your future.
- You may think about the positive changes cancer has created in your life. You may want to accept and adapt to those changes.

All of these responses are normal. But if the uncertainty is preventing you from enjoying life, or you have a lot of fear about it and feel overwhelmed, you should talk to a mental health professional about ways you can manage. Uncertainty may be a part of your life now but it doesn't have to affect your quality of life.

How Does Living with Uncertainty Affect Some Survivors?

Living with uncertainty can affect you in many different ways. It may cause you to feel upset or overwhelmed. It may motivate you to improve your life after cancer. There is no right or wrong way to feel about living with uncertainty; however, you can learn ways to manage.

Research has shown that some survivors experience depression, distress, and anxiety, and that these struggles can be related to living with uncertainty. Some people may tell you that you should just be happy that you survived, and that you shouldn't worry now. It's important to understand that living with uncertainty can be very difficult at times, and it's okay to talk about how it makes you feel.

While uncertainty about your health may lead you to worry, it may also motivate you to include more healthy behaviors in your lifestyle. You may choose to eat better, become more physically active to whatever extent possible and pay better attention to changes in your body. Feeling like you are doing something to promote good health may make you feel less uncertain about your future.

SOURCE: *Used with permission from the Lance Armstrong Foundation*

> We can never be absolutely certain that any woman is cured of
> breast cancer. Although we once spoke of a "cure" as 5 disease-free
> years after breast cancer was treated, we know now that breast
> cancer can recur 10 years or even 20 years later. So we think of
> "cure" as a retrospective term. It applies to women who don't
> experience a recurrence. For example more than 90% of women
> with ductal carcinoma in situ who are treated with surgery and
> radiation eventually die of other causes.
>
> —DR. SUSAN LOVE

Life after treatment is a complicated time of new hope and new
fear. It is a very common time for women to feel anxious and dis-
tressed, as the supports and the habits of treatment give way to a
return to "normal" life. Many women struggle with questions about
returning to work, about the changed nature of their relationships,
and with the lack of certainty about what the future holds. With the
realization that there's no certainty in your life, you're also more conscious of the value of the time you have right NOW.

Remission

The vagueness of the future prognosis can be unsettling, with words
like "remission" giving hope but no guarantee that the cancer will
never return. The term "remission" refers to the shrinking of cancer.
Complete remission means that the cancer is no longer detectable in
tests, scans, and X-rays. Complete remission might mean a cure;

however, in some cases the cancer can return. Partial remission refers to cancer that has shrunk but is still present. Partial remissions almost always return.

Quality of Life

Women who have undergone treatment for breast cancer should be reassured that their quality of life, once treatment has been completed, can be normal. Extensive studies have shown this. Women who have had chemotherapy may have a slight decrease in certain areas of function.

Some studies suggest that younger women, who represent about one fourth of breast cancer survivors, tend to have more problems adjusting to the stresses of breast cancer and its treatment. They have more psychosocial problems and trouble with emotional and social functioning. Some can feel isolated. Also, chemotherapy might have caused early menopause, which requires adjustment. There may also be sexual difficulties. All of which might need help with counseling and support groups directed to younger breast cancer survivors.

Living with Fear

The greatest fear for a woman who has had breast cancer is that the cancer will come back or spread. Learning to live with fear—and not allowing it to take over —is a challenge many women face.

Fear of recurrence has decreased a little with time, but still plagues me even two years after surgery and chemo. There's a funny phenomenon amongst us survivors where your mind automatically jumps to the worst

possible conclusion at the appearance of even the most innocuous symp-
toms. Even though rationally I know that in 99 percent of cases, an ache is
just an ache, there's a hypervigilance unique to survivorship that some-
times borders on hypochondria. We laugh about it in our support group
and we hope that our doctors don't think of us as too flaky. Generally, I
try to act only on unusual symptoms that last more than a several days,
but I figure increased vigilance is probably not such a bad thing overall.

Minimizing Risk

Many women feel an increased need to do everything they can in their
lives to minimize the risk of recurrence. Often, changes in lifestyle,
including quitting smoking, adopting a healthy diet, exercise, and an
increased emphasis on life/work balance become focal points for
breast cancer survivors returning to "normal" life after treatment.
Personal priorities also change—facing your own mortality can cause
you to reconsider relationships, patterns, and things that now seem
out of balance in your life.

Scientific studies increasingly support what many breast cancer
patients intuitively understand: that improving life habits can help us
lead longer, healthier lives. If you are overweight , it is a good idea to
lose weight. Although it is comforting to know that behavior modifica-
tion can reduce risk, there is no magic bullet and there are no
guarantees—the cancer could return in spite of doing everything
right—or conversely, the cancer might not return in spite of making
no changes at all. Do what you can to improve your chances, and don't
blame yourself if your cancer returns.

Exercise

Women who exercise more than three hours a week after being diagnosed with breast cancer might be able to lower their risk of recurrence and improve their chances of survival. Women with ER-positive breast cancer seem to get the most protective benefits from exercise. The equivalent of walking three to five hours a week at an average pace has the most benefit.

Low-Fat Diet

A low-fat diet (with about 25 percent of daily calories from fat) might reduce the risk of recurrence in postmenopausal women with ER-negative breast cancer. So far, there's no evidence of significant risk reduction for ER-positive cancers.

Stress

Another recent study suggests that stress might not be a factor in breast cancer recurrence. This contradicts an earlier study that suggested that major stress increased the likelihood of breast cancer coming back. That said, stress is still a significant quality-of-life issue, so it's important to find support and get help dealing with it even if it doesn't put you at higher risk for recurrence.

Will Your Daughters Have an Increased Risk of Breast or Other Cancers?

Because they are women, our daughters face the same overall risk for breast cancer as every woman faces. Other factors that could increase a daughter's risk include:

- How many first-degree (close) relatives have had breast, ovarian, or colon cancer?
- What age were you and/or the other relatives when diagnosed?
- Did breast cancer occur in one or both breasts?
- How old is your daughter?

Does your daughter have any other risk factors such as exposure to X-rays? If you are worried about hereditary breast cancer— breast cancer linked to the BRCA1 or BRCA2 gene—because of a strong family history, consider genetic counseling to estimate individual risk. However, it is important to keep the risk of hereditary breast cancer in perspective. This type of cancer accounts for only about 5 to 10 percent of all cases. Often there will be many family members affected over two to three generations and these people will often be diagnosed at an early age.

Our own experience of cancer will heighten our concern about the health of those we love. Again, good information can help reduce your anxiety and fears.

> It simply isn't possible to reduce the risk of recurrence to zero—to say positively that you are cured as of this moment and there is no chance you will have to worry about breast cancer again.
>
> —MUSA MAYER,
> *fourteen-year breast cancer survivor*

It is in the face of this uncertainty that women who have had a breast cancer diagnosis must live their lives. As Mayer writes, "My new companion was the unknown. I'd just have to find a way to live with it. It came with the territory."

SUMMARY

Breast cancer survivors experience a variety of short and long-term emotions and physical effects related to treatment, both positive and negative. These late effects can occur weeks, months, or years afterwards. Physical symptoms that occur later and may not be recognized as connected to original treatments include pain, numbness, and physical difficulties caused by surgery or scar tissue.

While sadness and depression are common, and it's realistic to have concerns about the future, many of us are grateful and often feel a sense of accomplishment; we find significant meaning from the experience and gain a new perspective on life.

On a positive note, survivors often say that cancer has forced them to stop taking their lives or their health for granted. As a result they focus on what is most meaningful and feel they are leading a better life after the diagnosis. Furthermore, they often want to share their experience with others. These people say that no matter what they've been through, no matter how harsh the treatments, they come away with something positive.

Recurrence

10

This chapter will help you understand your options if the cancer comes back

> To cure occasionally,
> to relieve often
> and to comfort, always.
>
> —ANONYMOUS, *sixteenth century*

What if the Cancer Comes Back?

When I first discovered I had breast cancer my surgeon said I had a 75 percent chance of recovery. When the cancer recurred, I knew I would make it again. I was put on tamoxifen and then Megace. Then, I was told my cancer was spreading. I am now having chemotherapy and I know it is helping me. My outlook is very positive.

Learning that the cancer is back is a terrible shock, and brings the same fear, anger, and pain as it did before. Your knowledge of the cancer care system and what happens during treatment are valuable, but knowing what's ahead may also leave you with a terrible feeling of dread. A recurrence is often more devastating or psychologically difficult for a woman than her initial diagnosis. Women who have recurrent breast cancer are encouraged to discuss their feelings with a counselor or therapist and consider joining a support group. Remember, you've traveled through cancer territory and faced its difficulties before. You can do it again.

TYPES OF RECURRENCE

There are three types of recurrent breast cancer: local, regional, and distant.

Local Recurrence

Local recurrence means that cancer cells remain in the original site, and over time, grow back. Local breast cancer recurrence is generally considered to result from the failure of the primary treatment to kill off all the original tumor cells. It is less common after mastectomy, but in rare cases can occur in the breast skin and fat that remains. In patients who have had a mastectomy, symptoms can be a lump or thickening on the chest wall, or a change in the feel of the skin. Local recurrence is more commonly a problem with breast-conserving surgery. Signs for such patients include lumps or thickening in the breast or armpit, changes in the breast, including skin changes (dimples or puckers in the breast), nipple discharge, scaling, inversion, and change in size, shape, color, or feel. Sometimes there is no sign on physical examination, but the local recurrence is seen on a mammogram. Local recurrences in women with implants occur most often in front of the implant, and with TRAM flap procedures, appear along the edge of the breast skin (not in the flap).

Regional Recurrence

Regional recurrence is more serious than local recurrence because it usually indicates that the cancer has spread beyond the breast. Regional breast cancer recurrences can occur in the chest muscles, in the lymph nodes under the breastbone or underarm, between the ribs, and above the collarbone around the neck. Symptoms can include hard lumps around the breast.

Distant Recurrence

Metastatic breast cancer to distant sites results from a few cells that have broken away from your breast and have traveled through the lymph system or bloodstream to a new site in your body. This recurrence is defined as the same type of cancer as the original. If, for example, it is in your liver, it is not liver cancer; it is breast cancer that has spread to your liver. The cancer is usually detected because of the symptoms, which can vary according to the area and extent of the metastatic disease. Also, the disease can be detected by follow-up diagnostics, such as chest X-ray or blood tests. Symptoms of metastatic breast cancer can include: pain in the back, hips, or sternum (metastases to the bones), shortness of breath or extreme fatigue (metastases to the lungs), loss of appetite, fatigue, yellow or itchy skin (liver metastases), or confusion, memory loss, headache and vision problems (brain metastases).

> I was devastated and traumatized by the original misdiagnosis. Chemotherapy in 1980 was truly dreadful, and I suffered with it for a full two years. In 1991, chemotherapy was much better due to effective antinauseants. I was thrilled to have the opportunity to have a bone marrow transplant, and the stress was worth it. My cancer has recurred once again and, except for being concerned about my children, who are suffering, I am living with it quite well.

Living with a Recurrence

> My first experience with cancer was twenty-seven years ago at age thirty-one. Emotionally, I went from one extreme to the other. The first time, nothing was going to get in my way. My second experience—a

mastectomy—was very sobering and brought me to a new level of
maturity and a new way of seeing myself in relation to the world
around me. The third or fourth time around I went into a year of
depression and anxiety, which produced my greatest learning experi-
ence: to face reality and take care of myself emotionally and physically.
When I emerged from this period, I made positive changes in my rela-
tionships and lifestyle. I kept a diary of my feelings, which taught me a
lot about myself when I was finally able to read it. I always thought it
could be helpful to share it with someone going through the same thing.
In some ways, this period of self-examination was worse than cancer.

Treatments for cancer recurrence are the same as the first occurrence: surgery, radiation, chemotherapy, and hormone therapy. Usually a woman with a local breast recurrence after breast-conserving surgery will undergo a mastectomy.

Researchers are currently studying new forms of chemotherapy and biological therapies. Your choice of treatment depends on what kind of treatments you had before, how much your cancer responds to hormones (its hormone receptor levels), how much time has passed between your first treatments and the recurrence, the site of recurrence, and whether or not you have gone through menopause.

The quality of life is still good. I'm a better person, more sensitive to oth-
ers, more understanding, kinder, and more loving. My spiritual life is
stronger and I have no fear of death, but I do want my suffering eased
as much as possible.

There are several drugs available to treat breast cancer recurrence. Some of them have been around longer than others and more is known about them. Aromatase inhibitors can be used if your tumor is estrogen receptor positive and you have not received one of these drugs before. Other chemotherapy drugs are doxorubicin (Adriamycin), epirubicin (Ellence), paclitaxel (Taxol), docetaxel (Taxotere), vinorelbine (Navelbine), and capecitabine (Xeloda). These drugs are used to treat metastatic disease. However, they are not a cure for breast cancer. Some women cannot tolerate these drugs at all, but for others it has improved their lives. If your tumor overexpresses Her2neu, trastuzumab (Herceptin) can be used. Other drugs presently being researched also show some promise for women with metastatic breast cancer. Ask your oncologist what he or she knows about these drugs and whether they might be appropriate for you.

Radiation can be used to relieve a very painful spot in the bone or chest wall. If you are having pain, there are very effective pain medications that can relieve your pain. Generally your family doctor or oncologist can advise you on this. However, if you are still having pain after seeking their advice, ask to see a pain specialist. Bisphosphonates (e.g., clodronate, pamidronate, and zoledronate) are used in women whose breast cancer has spread to the bones; the bisphosphonates will help strengthen bones and relieve pain.

What Are the Goals of Treatment for Metastatic Breast Cancer?

The goals of treatment for metastatic breast cancer are to reduce pain, relieve symptoms, and prolong survival as long as possible with as good a quality of life as possible. Although many women have benefited from treatment, which can prolong life in a way that is similar to treatment for other chronic diseases, doctors cannot and should not guarantee or predict promising results from treatment for metastatic disease. Length of life might be several years and it is impossible to predict what will happen to any particular individual. Again, mental well-being and learned coping skills can play a very important role in maintaining a sense of well-being. The support of family, friends, and support groups will also provide benefits.

Even with advanced disease and a poor prognosis, many cancer patients find hope by looking forward to planned events, like a child's graduation from high school or a gathering with friends. You may have work projects or hobbies that capture your attention and help relieve sadness and grief.

You may also find hope through your spirituality or religion. Cancer patients using a spiritual or religious basis for hope might believe that a higher power is helping them through the ups and downs of their disease, including being able to think about dying. You could find great help and comfort in talking with a spiritual leader or your clergyperson or by attending spiritual support groups.

You can use a more scientific or factual basis for hope, such as looking for information about treatments for advanced disease and clinical trials, getting additional opinions and surfing the Web for information.

People with cancer and their families usually combine many of these approaches to find hope. There is no right or wrong way to hope.

Explore a Variety of Ways to Release Your Feelings

There are many safe things you can do to release your feelings. You can:

♦ Tell your story of grief and loss several times to someone you trust, someone who listens to you without judgment. Each time you tell your story of loss, you release the feelings of grief associated with it.

- Express your feelings through a creative outlet you enjoy, such as music or art. Try banging on a piano, drumming, or scribbling with crayons.
- Have a good cry or, alternatively, a good, deep belly laugh. Watching a sad or funny movie that you enjoy can help trigger your tears or laughter.
- Find a safe place to yell or scream.
- Find a physical outlet, such as hitting pillows, going to a baseball batting cage or a golf driving range.
- Write down your thoughts and feelings in a journal.

> A distinction is made between "being cured" and "being healed." Healing, in the current vocabulary of serious illness, has more to do with finding of inner peace and coming to terms with our own mortality. In order to be healed, I think a person must take charge of as much of his or her life as the illness allows.
>
> —EVE COLEMAN, *Living, Dying and Cancer*

When a woman is facing a poor prognosis, she might understandably get very angry. The anger is often over caregivers ignoring the need for emotional support. Your relationship with your caregivers will very much depend on how comfortable you are talking about your fears, concerns, needs, and hopes. Be specific about what you expect from them. Let them know when you are in pain. Tell them you want to know about *all* the treatment options, and ask about clinical trials that might be under way at other treatment centers. You can also get help from the American Cancer Information Service (In the U.S.

1–800–422–6237) or the Canadian Cancer Society (1-888-939-3333). It is very important to maintain effective communication with your team of caregivers; they are on your side and will help you to make decisions and manage your care in the manner that *you* determine is best for you.

> The steps I took were the ways in which I took charge of my own life. While another person wouldn't necessarily do the things I did in order to begin the healing process, the important thing for any person, sick or well, is to be able to feel some measure of control over his or her life. We're all on a journey, and we're all at different stages of that journey.
>
> —EVE COLEMAN, *Living, Dying and Cancer*

When breast cancer is advanced to the point that death is expected, specialized end-of-life care is available to help. Expert teams provide hospice or palliative care to optimize independence, pain relief, dignity, and choices through the final and difficult period of dying.

> *Right now, I am having chemo for metastatic disease. I find it very difficult to take care of my two sons, paying for a sitter to take care of them. I'm very tired and at times very depressed and worried about dying and leaving my two little ones. My sex drive is non-existent, which puts a strain on my relationship with my husband, who is having lots of problems coping with living with someone who might die. It might be easier if there was more emotional support from the doctors. I was told my chemo might not work—period. No positive information at all. A support worker asked me if I wanted to know what it was like to die of lung cancer. Great support.*

Good listening skills and respect for what you and your family are experiencing can provide comfort and allow you to move through the stages of grief and anger that accompany a life-threatening prognosis. But many caregivers and family members are unable to provide the support needed. If so, the support can often be found in others within the family circle, friends, caregivers, and the community. The palliative care team, hospice program, or bereavement groups in your community can help you and those who care about you through this difficult time. They can help at any time during the progress of the disease, not just at the very end of life. Ask for help when you or someone you care about is suffering. No one needs to suffer alone or without good psychosocial support or pain management.

I don't think anyone will cure me, but my doctor helps me cope. And that means the world to me.

My journey of self-discovery and hope had taken me to places I thought I could no longer travel, both in the real and in the metaphoric sense. I had fought my way up rugged terrain, out of the pit which was clinical depression. Even though I teeter sometimes on the brink of that deep hole, occasionally losing my footing for a time, I try to remain on the high ground. My journey out was too difficult to chance the trip again.

As for more tangible trips, I had traveled to Boston and Maine with my family and my IV antibiotic bag. I had traveled, alone with my daughter Jennifer to the outer edges of Prince Edward Island and found peace as we drove our rental car around the island, going to the western cliffs of the remote Acadian country overlooking the ocean…Yes, I had traveled far.

—EVE COLEMAN, *Living, Dying and Cancer*

SUMMARY

Remember that, in the event of cancer recurrence, there are ways to help you cope with your fears and anxiety and to find hope, even when the disease has advanced and death is likely. You can gather information from your caregivers and from the sources listed in the Resources section of this book. You can contribute to your own care by using the coping and healing techniques that might have helped you in the past. You can call upon those counselors, friends, and family members who supported you in the past to help renew your strength and spirit.

HOPE

Hope is *an image of goals*
planted firmly in your mind.
When looking at life before you,
hope lines the paths you find.

Hope is a *well of courage*
nestled deep within your heart.
When faltering in fear and doubt,
hope pushes you to start.

Hope is an *urge to keep going*,
for limbs too tired and weak.
When apathy stills all desire,
hope sparks the fuel you seek.

Hope is a *promise of patience*
as you wait for distress to wane.
When all you can do is nothing,
hope pulls you through the pain.

Hope is *a spirit that lifts you*,
should heaviness pull at your soul.
When torn apart by losses,
hope mends to keep you whole.

—WENDY S. HARPHAM, M.D. *Happiness in a Storm*

When I learned that I was dying, that my life would no longer be
what it was, I could not imagine that I could have a life at all. I had
heard David's words when he told me I could stop living right
then—at the time of diagnosis—or live the rest of my life, but it
took time before the words made sense. Before the words made
sense, I sank to a very low point. That's when I went to "the land
of the living dead." I became not only sick in body, but also sick in
mind and spirit—depressed. Frederick Buechner seemed to be
speaking just to me in his book, Telling Secrets: A Memoir.
Buechner states, "...to lose track of our stories is to be profoundly
impoverished not only humanly but also spiritually." When I lost
my story, I lost the sense of who I was and what my life could be.
What had happened to me over the past months was beginning to
make sense. Only when I began to retell my story—by writing
about my past and by reinventing my present—was I able to live
with the specter of my unknown future. By finding my story
again, I was able pick up the threads of my life and recast it. I

could not regain life as I had known it, but I could regroup the resources which had served me well in my old life in order to move forward, out of the land of the living dead and toward a life of what some call "living with cancer," rather than "dying of cancer."

—EVE COLEMAN, *Living, Dying and Cancer*

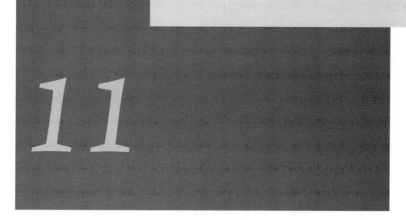

Advocates and Activists: Working Towards a Future without Cancer

11

This chapter discusses how and why people choose to become involved in cancer advocacy.

> The truth is, if you ask me to choose between winning the Tour de France and cancer, I would choose cancer. Odd as it sounds, I would rather have the title of cancer survivor than winner of the Tour, because of what it has done for me as a human being, a man, a husband, a son, and a father.
>
> —LANCE ARMSTRONG

This Isn't Fair!

You're right. It shouldn't have happened to you, or any of us, but it has. Maybe you've thought about giving up, about not fighting back. Most of us do at some point. But after the devastation and loneliness pass, when you're not so tired and miserable and sad, you will begin to think of life again. With time you will rediscover the opportunities that life can offer. You will make plans again.

> *A few years after my first diagnosis, I became involved in advocacy. My experience led me to believe that there were many things about the system that were broken, and that I could help others in my situation by adding a patient's perspective to the system change that is ongoing in cancer control. The work is very slow but very gratifying. For many of us advocates, I think it's our way of finding meaning from our cancer journey.*

Every woman who has had breast cancer is both activist and advocate; it's purely a matter of degree. Even the act of discussing and sharing triumphs and tragedies makes us advocates. A list of things that help for one woman will often get passed on to another, or sometimes, those tips and thoughts get turned into books—like this one!

For some women, recovery from breast cancer involves a desire to change the future—for ourselves and for our daughters and granddaughters. American and Canadian women know that public pressure can influence government commitments to critical health issues. Breast cancer activists have spoken out and made significant and positive changes in increased research funding, improved early-detection methods, primary prevention, and the involvement and influence of survivors in setting the research agenda and influencing all aspects of public policy in breast cancer.

As surely as scientific advances have changed how cancer is detected, treated, potentially prevented, and certainly studied, advocacy has changed the way we think about the role of the person with cancer in the medical process. Once thought of as a passive and grateful recipient in the treatment process, the cancer patient, or consumer—as we are now sometimes called—has evolved as an important and influential partner in all aspects of decision-making regarding cancer. As is true in most partnerships, the relationship between the advocacy and scientific communities has sometimes been one of excitement and success but at times has also seen the frustration of fundamental disagreement. While cancer advocacy has been a movement that has substantially changed the medical research process, even now it is frequently misunderstood.

> From the very beginning, advocates realized that if they were to have any real input into the decision-making processes related to cancer, they would have to be viewed as legitimate and respected members of the decision-making process. For that reason the advocate community is always demanding a "seat at the table."
>
> — EDISON LIU, ELEANOR NEALON, AND RICHARD KLAUSNER,
> *"Breast Disease 10 (5,6) (1998) 29-31IOS Press Perspective"*
> *from the National Cancer Institute (NCI)*

Some women choose to become activists after diagnosis and treatment, or after participating in a support group. For some women, an advocacy group is support—another way of making sense of the experience of surviving breast cancer. A diagnosis of breast cancer profoundly influences a woman's concerns about her future, and that of her daughters and other women she cares about. Activism can provide opportunities for women to make a difference. For women who were activists in the feminist movement or the environmental or consumer movements before their diagnosis, the progression to breast cancer activism may be natural and obvious. You can find contacts for advocacy groups in the U.S. and Canada in the Resources section of this book.

Roles for Advocates

1. **Advocate as researcher.** I have found that the presence of one or more advocates among scientists and physicians exerts a sobering, focusing and morally instructive influence. The best advocates also bring something else to the planning session. This is an original,

inquisitive, energetic view, sometimes enhanced by extensive experience in challenging fields other than science.

2. **The advocate as expert.** The simple answer is that the clinical scientists, even with years of experience, may still need help to see things from the patient perspective. Frankly, the value of this skill should be obvious. As anyone who has both coached and played sports would know, the game feels different from the sidelines. I have seen excellent scientists propose trials that ask questions of importance; nevertheless, they are doomed to failure because of their insensitivity to patients' concerns.

3. **The advocate as representative.** Some advocates provide valuable service representing little more than their own opinions and experience, but this is only part of the advocate's role. Advocates themselves have come to appreciate that their value is augmented by their willingness to be informed representatives of larger groups of patients.

4. **The advocate as advocate.** We must never forget there is still a need for contrary opinion, forceful critique, and even, on occasion, indignation. Advocates must stand their ground. Advocates must learn to join the fray without losing their viewpoints or their friends. This applies as well when advocates fight with each other! It is essential that the hard edge of advocacy still be felt when appropriate, lest all the accomplishments of the last few years dissipate in complacency or bitterness.

5. **All in all, I contend that the most important role for the advocate is advocate.** The researcher, the expert, and the representative are all secondary to the fighter for patients, rights, needs and dignity.

SOURCE: *Roles for Advocates: Breast Cancer Advocates in Clinical Research: A Trialist's Perspective,* by Larry Norton

SUMMARY

It is essential to recognize, however, that not all of us will choose to be activists. Some women will avoid it because it involves identifying with cancer. Most women try to forget about cancer as much as possible because they need to feel and be perceived as normal after a cancer diagnosis. Each of us must discover for ourselves what work and which relationships will make our lives meaningful. We must respect the choices each woman makes based on her life experiences, abilities, beliefs, and commitments. The most valued possession each of us has is time. How we choose to spend our time is up to each of us to determine.

Advocacy is indeed the completion of the comprehensive team. It is an expression of our unity of purpose as humans dedicated to the eradication of human suffering. It is the realization that we are all in this together.

—DR. LARRY NORTON,
Memorial Sloan-Kettering Cancer Center, New York

Glossary

ANESTHESIA: A drug or gas that is used to remove the feeling of pain. Local anesthesia involves the injection of a drug into a small area before a painful procedure, such as surgery. General anesthesia causes loss of consciousness.

AROMATASE INHIBITORS (AIS): Drugs called aromatase inhibitors (AIS) can help block the growth of estrogen-sensitive breast cancer tumors by lowering the amount of estrogen in the body. Estrogen is produced by the ovaries and other tissues of the body, using a substance called aromatase. AIS do not block estrogen production by the ovaries, but they can block other tissues from making this hormone. That's why AIS are used mostly in women who have reached menopause, when the ovaries are no longer producing estrogen. Currently, three AIS are approved by the U.S. Food and Drug Administration and Health Canada: anastrazole (Arimidex®), exemestane (Aromasin®), and letrozole (Femara®).

AXILLARY DISSECTION: Axilla is a term used for the armpit. An axillary dissection is surgery that removes some of the lymph nodes in the armpit.

BIOPSY: Removing tissue from some part of the body to study it more closely under a microscope for diagnosis.

BONE MARROW: The soft tissue that is found inside the bones. Red and white blood cells and platelets are produced in the bone marrow.

CARCINOGEN: Any substance that can cause cancer.

CAT SCAN: CAT stands for computerized axial tomography. This is a method of diagnosis that uses computers as well as X-rays. It can study tumors more closely than conventional X-rays.

CHEMOTHERAPY (CHEMO): Treatment that uses drugs to kill cancer cells. The drugs can be in the form of pills or injections.

DNA: Material present in living organisms that carries genetic information.

DUCT: A tube in the body that carries body fluids. In the breast, milk ducts carry milk from the lobule to the nipple. Sometimes cancer can develop in the milk ducts.

EDEMA: Excessive accumulation of fluid in tissue or body spaces.

ESTROGEN: Estrogen is produced by the ovaries and other tissues of the body, using a substance called aromatase. AIS do not block estrogen production by the ovaries, but they can block other tissues from making this hormone. That's why AIS are used mostly in women who have reached menopause, when the ovaries are no longer producing estrogen.

ESTROGEN RECEPTORS: Protein in cancer cells that bind to the female hormone estrogen.

GENES: Genes exist within cells in the body. They are the blueprint of the characteristics we inherit from our parents.

GRADE: A measure of how aggressive cancer cells look under a microscope. The more aggressive the cancer cells look, the more likely they are to spread to other parts of the body.

HER2/NEU: A gene that makes the human epidermal growth factor receptor 2 reaching breast cancer cells.

HORMONAL THERAPIES: This type of treatment can induce hormone production in the body or block hormone production. Hormone treatment for breast cancer usually involves blocking the production of the hormones estrogen and progesterone either by surgery that removes the ovaries, or by the use of specific drugs. Many breast tumors are "estrogen sensitive," meaning the hormone estrogen helps them to grow. Hormone treatment with drugs called aromatase inhibitors (AIS) can help block the growth of these tumors by lowering the amount of estrogen in the body.

HORMONES: Chemicals within the body that control growth, reproduction, sexual characteristics, and metabolism. Hormones are secreted into the blood and transported to specific organs (such as the breast).

IN SITU: In the natural or normal place. Cancer that is confined to the site of origin and is not invading neighboring tissue.

INVASIVE: A characteristic of malignant tumors, which invade and actively destroy surrounding tissue.

LOBULE: Lobes in the breast are divided into smaller structures called lobules. Milk is made in this part of the breast.

LUMPECTOMY: Surgery that removes the cancerous lump or tumor and a small amount of the normal breast tissue around it.

LYMPH: A body fluid that is similar to blood but does not have red blood cells. It transports white blood cells, called lymphocytes. The function of the lymph system is to provide fluid to body tissues and to carry waste away from the cells. Lymph flows through the body in the lymph vessels.

LYMPHEDEMA: A swelling of one of the limbs (arm, leg) as a result of the removal or radiation of the lymph nodes and lymph vessels in that limb. In women with breast cancer, this can occur in the arm or hand on the side that the surgery was done. It can occur anytime after surgery.

LYMPH NODES: Small lima-bean–shaped structures of the lymph system that act as filters.

MASTECTOMY: Surgery that removes the entire breast that is affected by cancer.

METASTASIS: The spread of cancer to another part of the body. The cancer cells are usually carried by the bloodstream or the lymphatic system. Plural: metastases.

MRI SCAN: MRI stands for magnetic resonance imaging. It is a technique that transmits radio waves through the body using a magnet and electric coil. It can provide more detailed information about tumors.

NECROSIS: Death of tissue in the body. This happens when not enough blood is supplied to the tissue, whether from diease, injury, radiation, or chemicals.

ONCOGENES: Genes that are capable of changing normal cells to cancer cells.

ONCOLOGIST: Oncology is the study of cancer, and an oncologist is a doctor who specializes in treating cancer patients.

OOPHORECTOMY: The surgical removal of one or both ovaries.

PATHOLOGIST: A doctor who specializes in examining body tissues. The pathologist determines if a disease is present.

PET SCAN: PET stands for position emission tomography. A scan that measures the activity or functional level of the brain.

PROGESTERONE: A female sex hormone involved in a number of functions, including menstruation and prenancy.

PROGNOSIS: An estimate of whether a disease (such as cancer) will stay the same or get worse in the future.

PROSTHESIS: An artificial substitute for a missing part of the body, such as a breast. For breast cancer patients, a breast form made of fabric or silicone that fits into the bra. A prosthesis can be used for both cosmetic or functional reasons (e.g., to ensure normal weight and balance to prevent sore shoulders or back problems).

PSYCHOSOCIAL ONCOLOGY: A complex word that means the field relating to the mind or the psyche, the "social" part of cancer having to do with the relationships people have with family and with society, and "oncology" meaning the branch of medicine that deals with cancer. Some hospitals and cancer centers refer to the field as "supportive care services" or "social work."

RADIATION THERAPY: High-energy radiation can be used to treat cancer by damaging and killing cancer cells. It is usually used after surgery if there is a risk that some cancer cells may have been left behind.

RADIOISOTOPES: Radioactive materials given to patients to make the organ that picks it up scannable.

SILICONE: A durable, synthetic substance that is used in some breast implants.

SYSTEMIC THERAPIES: Therapies that work throughout your blood system (such as chemotherapy). They may be recommended after your surgery or, in some cases, before. Also referred to as adjuvant systemic therapies, most involve anti-cancer medication (chemotherapy or hormone therapy) given after surgery to a woman who seems to be at high risk for a recurrence of her cancer.

TARGETED THERAPIES: Therapy (such as tamoxifen) that is targeted at a specific abnormality in breast cancer cells.

TUMOR MARKERS: Proteins that leak out of cancer cells and can be found in the blood. The most useful tumor markers for breast cancer are the CEA (carcinoembryonic antigen) and CA (cancer antigen) 15-3.

Resources

ONLINE DICTIONARIES

ADAM Health Illustrated Encyclopedia
(National Library of Medicine)
www.nlm.nih.gov/medlineplus/
encyclopedia.html

Celebrity Talking Dictionary
(BreastCancer.org)
www.breastcancer.org/dictionary/
welcome.html

Dana-Farber Cancer Institute Dictionary of Medical Terms
www.dana-farber.org/can/
dictionary

Dictionary of Cancer Terms
(National Cancer Institute)
www.cancer.gov/dictionary

Medical Dictionary
(Aetna InteliHealth)
www.intelihealth.com

Medical Dictionaries and Glossaries in Nine European Languages
(Martindale's Health Science Guide 2000)
allserv.rug.ac.be

Talking Glossary of Genetic Terms
(National Human Genome Research Institute)
www.genome.gov

RESOURCE SITES: CANADA

Canadian Breast Cancer Network
Toll -free: 1-800-685-8820
In Ottawa: (613) 230-3044
www.cbcn.ca

Canadian Breast Cancer Society
Toll-free: 1-800-567-8767
Local: (519)-336-0746
www.bcsc.ca

Canadian Cancer Society
Toll-free: 1-888-939-3333
www.cancer.ca

Canadian Breast Cancer Foundation
In Toronto: (416) 596-6773
Toll-free: 1-800-387-9816
www.cbcf.org

L'auto-examen des seins (AES)
www.examendusein.ca (français)
www.breastselfexam.ca (English)

Willow Breast Cancer Support and Resource Services
Toll-free: 1-888-778-3100
In Toronto: (416) 778-5000
www.willow.org

ADVOCACY

Cancer Advocacy Coalition of Canada
www.canceradvocacycoalition.
com

Campaign to Control Cancer (C2CC)
www.controlcancer.ca

National Cancer Leadership Forum
www.cancerforum.ca

RESOURCE SITES: UNITED STATES, GENERAL

American Cancer Society
www.cancer.org

American Institute for Cancer Research (AICR)
www.aicr.org

Asian American Health
www.baylor.edu/~Charles_Kemp/
asian_health.html

Association of Cancer Online Resources
www.acor.org

Association of Community Cancer Centers (ACCC)
www.accc-cancer.org

Black Health Net
www.blackhealthnetwork.com

Cancer Care Inc.
www.cancercare.org

Cancer411.org
www.cancer411.org

Cancer Guide
www.cancerguide.org

Cancer Hope Network
www.cancerhopenetwork.org

Cancer Information and Counseling Line (CICL)
www.amc.org/html/info/h_info_
cicl.html

Cancer News on the Net
www.cancernews.com

CancerQuilt
www.thequilt.com

Cancer Research Foundation of America (CRFA)
www.preventcancer.org

Centers for Disease Control and Prevention (CDC)
www.cdc.gov

Center for Mind-Body Medicine
www.cmbm.org

Center to Advance Palliative Care (CAPC)
www.capcmssm.org

Cycle of Hope
www.cycleofhope.org

FDA Cancer Liaison Program
http://cdmrp.army.mil/bcrp/

Find Cancer Experts
www.FindCancerExperts.com

Gay Health
www.gayhealth.com

The Intercultural Cancer Council (ICC)
www.icc.bcm.tmc.edu

Lance Armstrong Foundation
www.laf.org

The Lesbian Community Cancer Project
www.lccp.org

The Mautner Project for Lesbians with Cancer
www.mautnerproject.org

National Asian Women's Health Organization
www.nawho.org

National Cancer Institute (NCI)
www.nci.nih.gov

National Center for Complementary and Alternative Medicine (NCCAM)
www.nccam.nih.gov

National Coalition for Cancer Survivorship (NCCS)
www.cansearch.org

National Comprehensive Cancer Network (NCCN)
www.nccn.org

National Hospice and Palliative Care Organization (NHPCO)
www.nhpcao.org

National Self-Help Clearinghouse
www.selfhelpweb.org

Native American Cancer Research
natamcancer.org

Office of Cancer Survivorship
dccps.nci.nih.gov/ocs/about.html

The Office of Minority Health
www.omhrc.gov

OncoLink
www.oncolink.upenn.edu

Patient Advocate Foundation
www.patientadvocate.org

The Wellness Community
www.wellness-community.org

RESOURCE SITES: UNITED STATES, SPECIFIC

American Society for Clinical Oncology
www.asco.org

Avon's Breast Cancer Awareness Crusade
http://www.avoncompany.com/women/avoncrusade/

Breast Cancer.Net
www.breastcancer.net/

Cancerfact.Com
www.cancerfacts.com

Department of Defense Breast Cancer Decision Guide
www.bcdg.org

Fertile Hope
www.fertilehope.org

Inflammatory Breast Cancer Help Page
www.ibcsupport.org

Living Beyond Breast Cancer
www.lbbc.org

Male Breast Cancer Information Center
http://www.cancer.gov/cancerinfo/pdq/treatment/malebreast/Patient

Mothers Supporting Daughters with Breast Cancer (MSDBC)
www.mothersdaughters.org

National Alliance of Breast Cancer Organizations (NABCO)
www.nabco.org

National Breast Cancer Coalition
www.stopbreastcancer.org

National Cancer Institute
www.cancer.gov

National Comprehensive Cancer Network
www.nccn.org

National Lymphedema Network
www.lymphnet.org

Oncolink
Abramson Cancer Center of the University of Pennsylvania
www.oncolink.org

Patient Advocate Foundation
www.patientadvocate.org

Susan G. Komen Breast Cancer Foundation
www.Komen.org

Susan Love MD
www.susanlovemd.org

Y-ME National Breast Cancer Association
www.y-me.org

BOOKS

Bazell, Robert. HER-2: The Making of Herceptin, a Revolutionary Treatment for Breast Cancer. New York: Random House, 1998.

Chan, David, John Glaspy, and Frank Stockdale. Breast Cancer: Real Questions, Real Answers. New York: Marlowe & Company, 2006.

Cohen, Deborah, and Robert Geldfand, MD Just Get Me Through This: The Practical Guide to Breast Cancer. New York: Kensington Publishing, 2001.

Gelman, Dr. Karen, Dr. David McCready, and Dr. Ivo Olivotto. The Intelligent Patient Guide to Breast Cancer: All You Need to Know to Take an Active Part in Your Treatment, 4th ed. Intelligent Patient Guide Ltd., 2006.

Glacel, Barbara Pate. *Hitting The Wall: Memoir of a Cancer Journey.* Veedersburg, IN: Hara Publishing, 2001.

Hirshaut, Yashar, and Peter Pressman MD *Breast Cancer: The Complete Guide.* New York: Bantam, 2004.

Keon, Joseph. *The Truth About Breast Cancer: A 7-Step Prevention Plan.* Larkspur, CA: Parissound, 1998.

Link, John, Cynthia Forsthoff, and James Waisman. *The Breast Cancer Survival Manual: A Step-by-Step Guide for the Woman with Newly Diagnosed Breast Cancer,* 3rd ed. New York: Owl Books, 2003.

Love, Dr. Susan M., and Karen Lindsey. *Dr. Susan Love's Breast Book,* 4th ed. Cambridge, Da Capo Lifelong Books, 2005.

Mayer, Musa. *Advanced Breast Cancer: A Guide to Living with Metastatic Disease,* 2nd ed. Cambridge, O'Reilly, 1998.

Silver, Marc. *Breast Cancer Husband: How to Help Your Wife (and Yourself) during Diagnosis, Treatment and Beyond.* New York: Rodale Books, 2004.

Steligo, Kathy. *The Breast Reconstruction Guidebook,* 2nd ed. San Carlos, CA: Carlo Press, 2005.

Weiss, Marisa. *Living Beyond Breast Cancer: A Survivor's Guide for When Treatment Ends and the Rest of Your Life Begins.* New York: Random House, 1998.

NUTRITION

Dyer, Diana. *A Dietitian's Cancer Story: Information & Inspiration for Recovery & Healing From a 3-Time Cancer Survivor.* Dexter, MI: Swan Press, 2000.

Errey, Sally, and Trevor Simpson. *Staying Alive! Cookbook for Cancer Free Living: Real Survivors, Real Recipes, Real Results.* Vancouver: Belissimo Books, 2004.

Harvard Medical School. *Healthy Eating: A Guide to the New Nutrition.* Boston: Harvard Medical School, 2003.

Quillin, Patrick, and Noreen Quillin. *Beating Cancer with Nutrition.* Tulsa, OK: Nutrition Times Press, 2001.

SPIRITUALITY

Buechner, Frederick. *Telling Sercets: A Memoir.* San Francisco: HarperSanFrancisco, 1992.

Frank, Arthur. *At the Will of the Body: Reflections on Illness.* New York: Houghton Mifflin Company, 1991.

———. *The Wounded Storyteller: Body, Illness, and Ethics.* Chicago: University of Chicago Press, 1995.

Himes, Mavis. *The Sacred Body: A Therapist's Journey.* Toronto: Stoddart. 2002.

Kuner, Susan, et al. *Speak the Language of Healing: Living with Breast Cancer without Going to War.* San Francisco: Conari Press, 1999.

PARTNERS

Fincannon, Joy L., and Katherine V. Bruss. *Couples Confronting Cancer: Keeping Your Relationship Strong.* American Cancer Society, 2002.

Halpin, Brendan. *It Takes a Worried Man: A Memoir.* New York: Random House, 2003.

Silver, Marc. *Breast Cancer Husband: How to Help Your Wife (and Yourself) during Diagnosis, Treatment and Beyond.* New York: Rodale Books, 2004.

CHILDREN

Harpham, Wendy S. *When a Parent Has Cancer: A Guide to Caring for Your Children.* New York: HarperCollins, 2004.

Heiney, Susan P., Joan Hermann, et al. *Cancer in the Family: Helping Children Cope with a Parent's Illness.* American Cancer Society, 2001.

McCue, Kathleen, and Ron Bonn. *How to Help Children through a Parent's Serious Illness.* New York: St. Martin's Press, 1996.

COMPLEMENTARY THERAPIES

American Cancer Society. *Complementary and Alternative Cancer Methods.* American Cancer Society, 2000.

Bognar, David. *Cancer: Increasing Your Odds for Survival: A Resource Guide for Integrating Mainstream, Alternative and Complementary Therapies.* Alameda, CA: Hunter House, 1998.

Geffen, Jeremy R., MD. *The Journey Through Cancer: An Oncologist's Seven-Level Program for Healing and Transforming the Whole Person.* New York: Three Rivers Press, 2000.

Kaur, Sat Dharam. *A Call to Women: The Healthy Breast Program & Workbook: A Naturopathic Guide to Preventing Breast Cancer.* Kingston, ON: Quarry Health Books, 2000.

Labriola, Dan, ND. *Complementary Cancer Therapies: Combining Traditional and Non-Traditional Therapies.* Roseville, CA: Prima Health, 2000.

Williams, Penelope. *Alternatives in Cancer Therapy: The Case for Choice.* Toronto: Key Porter Books, 2000.

———. *Breast Cancer: Landscape of an Illness.* Toronto: Penguin Canada, 2004.

EMOTIONAL SUPPORT

Armstrong, Lance, and Sally Jenkins. *It's Not about the Bike: My Journey Back to Life.* New York: Penguin, 2000.

Cohen, Deborah, and Robert Geldfand, MD. *Just Get Me Through This: The Practical Guide to Breast Cancer.* New York: Kensington Publishing Corporation, 2001.

Cunningham, Alastair J. *The Healing Journey: Overcoming the Crisis of Cancer.* Toronto: Key Porter Books, 2000.

Geffen, Jeremy R., MD. *The Journey Through Cancer: An Oncologist's Seven-Level Program for Healing and Transforming the Whole Person.* New York: Three Rivers Press, 2000.

Glacel, Barbara Pate. *Hitting the Wall: Memoir of a Cancer Journey.* Veedersburg, IN: Hara Publishing, 2001.

Harham, Wendy S. *Happiness in a Storm: Facing Illness and Embracing Life as a Healthy Survivor.* New York: W.W. Norton, 2005.

Kapusta, Beth, Canadian Association of Psychosocial Oncology (CAPO), and TransCanada Pipelines. *The Emotional Facts of Life with Cancer: A Guide to Counselling and Support for Patients, Families and Friends.* Toronto, ON: CAPO, 2003. Available online at http://www.capo.ca/docs/bookletREVISED.pdf or from CCS 1-888-939-3333.

Peltosaari, Leila. *Dancing with Fear: Tips and Wisdom from Breast Cancer Survivors.* Verdun, QC: Tikka Books, 2005.

Weiss, Marisa, and Ellen Weiss. *Living Beyond Breast Cancer: A Survivor's Guide for When Treatment Ends and the Rest of Your Life Begins.* New York: Three Rivers Press, 1998.

RECONSTRUCTION

Berger, Karen, and John Bostwick. *A Woman's Decision: Breast Care, Treatment & Reconstruction.* New York: St. Martin's Griffin, 1998.

Steligo, Kathy. *The Breast Reconstruction Guidebook*, 2nd ed. San Carlos, CA: Carlo Press, 2005.

METASTATIC DISEASE

Mayer, Musa. *Advanced Breast Cancer: A Guide to Living with Metastatic Disease*, 2nd ed. Cambridge: O'Reilly, 1998.

PREVENTION

Keon, Joseph. *The Truth About Breast Cancer: A 7-Step Prevention Plan.* Larkspur, CA: Parissound, 1998.

With thanks to Carol Burnham Cook of Willow for her help with the bibliography and resources section of this book.

SUPPORT GROUP DEVELOPMENT

Kelly, Pat. *Leadership from the Heart.* Toronto: Key Porter Books, 2000.

Index